DR. EARL MINDELL'S
Natural
REMEDIES FOR 150 AILMENTS

EARL MINDELL
R.Ph., Ph.D.

Basic Health
PUBLICATIONS, INC.

The information contained in this book is based upon the research and personal and professional experiences of the author. It is not intended as a substitute for consulting with your physician or other healthcare provider. Any attempt to diagnose and treat an illness should be done under the direction of a healthcare professional.

The publisher does not advocate the use of any particular healthcare protocol but believes the information in this book should be available to the public. The publisher and author are not responsible for any adverse effects or consequences resulting from the use of the suggestions, preparations, or procedures discussed in this book. Should the reader have any questions concerning the appropriateness of any procedures or preparation mentioned, the author and the publisher strongly suggest consulting a professional healthcare advisor.

Basic Health Publications, Inc.
8200 Boulevard East • North Bergen, NJ 07047 • 1-201-868-8336

Library of Congress Cataloging-in-Publication Data
Mindell, Earl.
  [Natural remedies for 150 ailments]
  Dr. Earl Mindell's natural remedies for 150 ailments / Earl Mindell.—
New updated & expanded.
    p. cm.
  Includes bibliographical references and index.
  ISBN 1-59120-118-7
  1. Naturopathy. 2. Dietary supplements. 3. Herbs—Therapeutic use.
  4. Medicine, Popular. I. Title: Doctor Earl Mindell's natural remedies for
150 ailments. II. Mindell, Earl. Natural remedies for 101 ailments. III. Title.

  RZ440.M5385   2004
  615.5'35—dc22   2004015076

Editor: Carol Rosenberg and Christopher Mariadason
Typesetting: Gary Rosenberg and Theresa Wiscovitch
Cover design: Mike Stromberg

Printed in Canada

10 9 8 7 6 5 4 3 2

Contents

THERAPIES

Preface

Congratulations! By opening this book, you have taken a giant step toward better health and greater vitality for the rest of your life.

Because I am a pharmacist as well as a nutritionist and herbalist, I have a unique point of view on natural and alternative health. I have firsthand knowledge of how drugs work in the body, how they are prescribed, and why doctors prescribe them. I can tell you that the best thing you can do for your health is avoid prescription and over-the-counter drugs and turn to natural remedies to relieve whatever ails you.

The real secret to fabulous good health well into old age has a lot to do with common sense and moderation. If you put water in your car's gas tank, your car will break down. Doesn't it make sense that if you eat a lot of junk food and often drink sugary beverages that your body is going to break down? If you follow some very simple basic guidelines for a healthy lifestyle, you will find many of your chronic ailments vanishing. And you'll be surprised at how easy and how rewarding it is!

That's why I created my favorite natural remedies for 150 common ailments. These recipes will show you how your body can use all the wonderful natural remedies and preventive strategies to keep it running in top condition. I hope you turn to this book many times to find valuable information in your search for living a healthy and pain-free life.

Stay healthy!

Earl Mindell, R.Ph., Ph.D.

**For a list of other books by Dr. Earl Mindell,
visit http://www.DrEarlMindell.com.**

Introduction

Natural Remedies for Your Medicine Cabinet

It wasn't so long ago that white willow bark was prescribed for pain, and chamomile tea for stomach aches. Today, herbal remedies such as these have completely disappeared from mainstream medicine. The pharmaceutical industry has learned how to take natural substances and transform their health-promoting constituents into synthetic versions, which have become our prescription and over-the-counter drugs. While these synthetic drugs have advanced medicine in some cases, they have done so with great expense, debilitating side effects, and interactive complications.

Lately, we've been relearning that Mother Nature really knows how to package remedies so that they are safe and effective. Once again, millions of people are turning to gentler yet effective means for curing all types of health conditions. This book features Dr. Mindell's favorite natural remedies for 150 common ailments. In these pages, this world-renowned health expert provides you with hundreds of natural time-tested remedies for whatever ails you.

Learn how you can use natural remedies to replace many of the most commonly used over-the-counter drugs in the treatment of the following ailments:

- Allergies
- Arthritis Pain
- Cardiovascular Disease
- Cholesterol
- Colds and Flu
- Depression
- Diabetes
- Headaches

- Indigestion
- Nausea
- Osteoporosis
- PMS
- Premature Aging
- Prostate Disorders
- Skin Problems
- Weight Loss

and more!

You'll find yourself turning to this book many times to find valuable information in your search for living a healthy, natural, and pain-free life.

A Note about Dosages

The dosage recommendations for the supplements and herbs listed in this book are for adults. For children between ages six and twelve, half of the adult dosage should be sufficient. For children under age six, always seek the guidance of a healthcare professional before administering any kind of supplement.

The herbs listed in this book can be taken in capsule form as directed on the label. When purchasing herbs in capsule form, look for the words "standardized herbal extract" on the label. Herbal teas are also available, but they are weaker than the standardized herbal extracts. Other herbal products should be used only topically. Their labels will state "for external use only."

The herbs and supplements recommended for each disorder can be taken together. In many cases, a remedy will have to be continued for at least thirty days before results are seen.

CAUTION: If you are pregnant or nursing, consult your healthcare professional before using any of these remedies.

Acne

Acne is an inflammatory skin disorder of the face, back, and chest. Although it is usually associated with hormone fluctuations during puberty, it can and does affect many adults. Whiteheads, blackheads, and pimples, which are characteristics of acne, result from an overgrowth of bacteria in oil-clogged pores. Although keeping the skin clean is very important in helping to control acne, it is not enough. Vitamins, minerals, and herbal supplements, as well as healthy eating and exercise habits, can be very beneficial.

SUPPLEMENTS

- Chromium: 200–600 mg daily.
- Selenium: 100–200 mcg daily.
- Vitamin A: 5,000–10,000 IU daily.
- Vitamin C: 500–1,000 mg with 500 mg of bioflavonoids daily.
- Vitamin E: 400–500 IU daily.
- Zinc: 15 mg of elemental zinc (read label), once or twice daily.

HERBS

- Echinacea: as directed on label.
- Goldenseal: as directed on label.

CONSIDER / TRY TO

- Aerobic exercise.
- Detoxification (see TOXICITY on page 280).
- Drink six to eight glasses of pure water daily.
- Eat more raw vegetables.
- Eat yogurt with live cultures.

AVOID / WATCH OUT FOR

- High-fat foods and other junk foods.
- Refined carbohydrates.
- Stress.
- Sugar, caffeine, and chocolate.

ADD/ADHD

Attention deficit disorder (ADD) is a condition characterized by a short or poor attention span and inappropriate, impulsive behavior. Attention deficit hyperactivity disorder (ADHD) is ADD with hyperactivity. These disorders usually affect school-aged children, but may continue into adulthood. Symptoms include fidgeting, excessive talking, disregard of consequences, and an inability to concentrate. Psychostimulant drugs are often prescribed to control ADD/ADHD, but natural remedies, including nutritional supplements and exercise, offer nonprescription alternatives.

SUPPLEMENTS

- Calcium: 500–1,000 mg daily (older women: 1,500–2,000 mg).
- Magnesium: 250–500 mg daily.
- MSM: 1,000 mg, one to three times daily.

HERBS

- Bacopa extract: 100 mg daily.
- Club moss (Huperzine A): as directed on label.
- Ginkgo biloba extract: 60 mg, one to three times daily.
- Grape seed/green tea complex: 100 mg of each, twice daily.
- Green tea extract: 100 mg, twice daily.
- Phosphatidylserine (PS): 300–600 mg daily.
- St. John's wort (dual action): 300 mg, once or twice daily.

CONSIDER / TRY TO

- Allergy elimination diet.
- Biofeedback.
- Exercise regularly.

AVOID / WATCH OUT FOR

- Dairy products.
- Junk foods.
- Refined carbohydrates.
- Stress.

Alcohol Abuse/Alcoholism

An occasional alcoholic beverage is enjoyed by many adults. However, when indulging in alcohol becomes a frequent occurrence or when alcohol is consumed to excess even only occasionally, it constitutes alcohol abuse. Alcohol abuse can lead to alcoholism in susceptible people. Both alcohol abuse and alcoholism can interfere with work, relationships, and socialization. Willpower, along with natural remedies, can start anyone with this destructive problem on the road to sobriety.

ALCOHOL ABUSE/ALCOHOLISM

SUPPLEMENTS

- Calcium: 500–1,000 mg daily (older women: 1,500–2,000 mg).
- Glutathione: 50 mg, one to three times daily.
- MSM: 1,000 mg, one to three times daily.
- Vitamin B complex: 25–50 mg daily.
- Vitamin B_1 (thiamin): 50–500 mg daily.
- Vitamin C: 500–1,000 mg daily.

HERBS

- Chamomile: as directed on label.
- Ginger root extract: as directed on label.
- Kudzu capsules: 500–1,500 mg daily (as capsules).
- Milk thistle (silymarin): 140 mg, one to three times daily (as capules).
- Turmeric: as directed on label.

CONSIDER / TRY TO

- Drink six to eight glasses of pure water daily.
- Drink a few cups of herbal tea, such as chamomile, throughout the day.

AVOID / WATCH OUT FOR

- Cough syrups that contain alcohol.
- Mouthwashes that contain alcohol.

Allergies to Dust, Mold, and Dander

Allergic reactions are the immune system's response to perceived invaders in the body, such as mold or dust. These invaders, which are usually harmless, are known as allergens. An allergic reaction can range anywhere from mild to severe. Mild symptoms include itchy, watery eyes and sneezing. A severe reaction can affect respiratory and circulatory function. For mild cases and to reduce the frequency of attacks, nutritional supplements and other natural remedies can provide relief. See also HAY FEVER.

ALLERGIES TO DUST, MOLD, AND DANDER

SUPPLEMENTS

- Digestive enzymes: one to three capsules with each meal.
- Magnesium: 250–500 mg daily.
- MSM: 1,000 mg, one to three times daily.
- Omega-3 fatty acids: 50 mg, one to three times daily (as fish oil capsules).
- Vitamin B complex: 25–50 mg daily.
- Vitamin C: 500–1,000 mg daily.
- Zinc: 15 mg of elemental zinc (read label), once or twice daily.

HERBS

- Borage oil: 500–1,000 mg daily (as capsules) *or* evening primrose oil: 500–1,000 mg daily (as capsules).
- Echinacea: as directed on label.
- Ginkgo biloba extract: 60 mg, one to three times daily.
- Grape seed extract (PCOs): 100 mg, one to three times daily.
- Licorice root: 450 mg, one to three times daily (as capsules).
- Quercetin: 400 mg before eating, one to three times daily.

CONSIDER / TRY TO

- A colon-cleansing program.
- Detoxification (see Toxicity on page 280).
- Drink six to eight glasses of pure water daily.
- Immune-system boosters (see Immune System, Weakened on page 164).

AVOID / WATCH OUT FOR

- Excessive dust in bedroom.
- Pets in bedroom.

Allergies to Food

A food allergy is an allergic reaction to a certain food, such as milk, shellfish, nuts, chocolate, or soy, or food additives, such as preservatives and colorings. Symptoms may include mild to severe skin rash, hives, gastrointestinal upset, and/or shortness of breath. Severe reactions can be life threatening. A person with a food allergy must eliminate the offending food from his or her diet, but may find natural remedies helpful in reducing the severity of symptoms in the event the food is accidentally consumed.

SUPPLEMENTS

- Digestive enzymes: one to three capsules with each meal.
- Glutamine: 50–150 mg daily.
- Magnesium: 250–500 mg daily.
- MSM: 1,000 mg, one to three times daily.
- Vitamin B complex: 25–50 mg daily.
- Zinc: 15 mg of elemental zinc (read label), once or twice daily.

HERBS

- Borage oil: 500–1,000 mg daily (as capsules) *or* evening primrose oil: 500–1,000 mg daily (as capsules).
- Goldenseal: as directed on label.
- Licorice root: 450 mg, one to three times daily (as capsules).

CONSIDER / TRY TO

- Allergy elimination diet.
- Colon-cleansing program.
- Detoxification (see TOXICITY on page 280).
- Drink six to eight glasses of pure water daily.

AVOID / WATCH OUT FOR

- Excessive alcohol consumption.
- Food dyes, preservatives, and other additives.
- Foods known to cause an allergic reaction.
- Stress.

Alzheimer's Disease

Alzheimer's disease is the most common cause of dementia—a progressive decline in mental ability. It is often associated with old age, but can occur as early as middle age. The cause of Alzheimer's disease is unknown. Symptoms include loss of short-term memory, personality changes, and diminished ability to recognize people, places, and things. Although Alzheimer's disease is currently incurable, natural remedies can provide some benefit. See also MEMORY LOSS; SENILE DEMENTIA.

SUPPLEMENTS

- Coenzyme Q_{10}: 60 mg, one to three times daily.
- L-Carnitine: 50–500 mg daily.
- Magnesium: 250–500 mg daily.
- Melatonin: 1–3 mg, just before bedtime.
- Phosphatidylserine (PS): 300–600 mg daily.
- Pregnenolone: 10 mg daily.
- Vitamin B complex: 25–50 mg daily.
- Zinc: 15 mg of elemental zinc (read label), once or twice daily.

HERBS

- Bacopa extract: as directed on label.
- Club moss (Huperzine A): as directed on label.
- Ginkgo biloba extract: 60 mg, one to three times daily.
- Grape seed/green tea complex: 100 mg of each twice daily.

AVOID / WATCH OUT FOR

- Aluminum foil and cookware (high aluminum absorption may be linked to Alzheimer's disease).

Anemia

In anemia, either the number of red blood cells or the amount of hemoglobin (oxygen-carrying protein) in the red blood cells is inadequate for an ample supply of oxygen to reach the body systems. Common causes of anemia are excessive bleeding, decreased red blood cell production, and increased red blood cell destruction. Symptoms vary, but may include fatigue, weakness, and lightheadedness. Supplementing with certain vitamins, minerals, and herbs can aid the body's production of red blood cells.

SUPPLEMENTS

- Folic acid: 400–800 mcg daily.
- Iron (organic): 10–15 mg of essential iron daily.
- Vitamin B_{12}: 100–1,000 mcg daily.
- Vitamin C: 500–1,000 mg daily.

HERBS

- Chive: as directed on label.
- Dong quai: as directed on label.
- Quinoa: as directed on label.
- Rose hip: as directed on label.
- Watercress: as directed on label.

AVOID / WATCH OUT FOR

- Burdock root and yellow dock interfere with iron absorption.
- Excessive consumption of coffee and caffeinated soft drinks.
- Too much iron (that is, two to five times more than the RDA).

Angina

Angina is temporary pain or feeling of pressure
in the chest due to a lack of adequate oxygen
to the heart muscle. The most common cause
of angina is coronary artery disease—a condition
in which blood flow in the coronary artery is
obstructed by fatty deposits. The pain or
discomfort usually lasts for only a few minutes
and is often triggered by physical activity. The
underlying condition should be treated or,
more preferably, prevented. Natural remedies,
such as nutritional supplementation and certain
lifestyle changes, can be helpful.

SUPPLEMENTS

- Carnitine: 50–500 mg daily.
- Coenzyme Q_{10}: 60 mg, one to three times daily.
- Magnesium: 250–500 mg daily.
- Soy isoflavonoids: 40–60 mg daily.
- Vitamin E: 400–500 IU daily.

HERBS

- Cayenne: as directed on label.
- Dandelion: as directed on label.
- Garlic: 500 mg daily.
- Ginseng: as directed on label.
- Hawthorne extract: as directed on label.

CONSIDER / TRY TO

- Aerobic exercise.
- Eat fiber-rich foods.
- Eat foods that contain essential fatty acids.
- Eat more raw fruits and vegetables.
- Lose weight if necessary.

AVOID / WATCH OUT FOR

- Alcohol.
- All stimulants, including caffeine.
- Salt and sugar.
- Saturated fats.
- Smoking.
- Spicy foods and fried foods.
- Stress.

Anxiety

Everyone experiences some level of anxiety—a
sense of apprehension or fear—at one time or
another during the course of his or her life. It is
a normal response to stress. Feelings of anxiety
can range in intensity and can last for any
length of time. An anxiety disorder is
characterized by excessive, extreme, or
unrealistic persistent worry about any number
of things or activities. Certain herbs can reduce
anxious feelings almost immediately. Other
supplements and lifestyle changes can help,
as well.

SUPPLEMENTS

- Calcium: 500–1,000 mg daily (older women: 1,500–2,000 mg).
- Inositol hexanicotinate (no-flush niacin): 250–500 mg daily.
- Magnesium: 250–500 mg daily.
- Multi–trace mineral formula: as directed on label.
- Vitamin B complex: 25–50 mg.
- Zinc: 15 mg of elemental zinc (read label), once or twice daily.

HERBS

- Chamomile: as directed on label.
- Hops: as directed on label.
- Skullcap: as directed on label.
- St. John's wort (dual action): 300 mg, once or twice daily.
- Valerian: as directed on label.

CONSIDER / TRY TO

- Exercise regularly.
- Meditation and/or yoga.

AVOID / WATCH OUT FOR

- Aspartame.
- Caffeine.
- Monosodium glutamate (MSG).
- Refined carbohydrates.
- Stress.
- Sugar.

Appetite Loss

Any number of conditions can trigger a loss of appetite, including pinworms, gastrointestinal problems, tick bite, strep throat, hepatitis, and depression. It's a good idea to determine and treat the underlying cause whenever possible. Some nutritional supplements can stimulate the appetite, as can eating certain seeds and whole grains. Be aware that some prescription drugs can affect the sense of taste, which may result in a reluctance to eat. If this is the case, look into a natural alternative.

SUPPLEMENTS

- Biotin: 300 mcg daily.
- Calcium: 500–1,000 mg daily (older women: 1,500–2,000 mg).
- Copper: 2–3 mg daily.
- Magnesium: 250–500 mg daily.
- Vitamin A: 5,000–10,000 IU daily.
- Vitamin B complex: 25–50 mg daily.
- Vitamin B_1 (thiamin): 50–500 mg daily.
- Zinc: 15 mg of elemental zinc (read label), once or twice daily.

HERBS

- Black currant: drink as tea.
- Cayenne: as directed on label.
- Fennel: as directed on label.

CONSIDER / TRY TO

- Eat more protein and whole grains.
- Eat pumpkin seeds and sunflower seeds.
- Sprinkle one tablespoon of brewer's yeast over food or dissolve in a beverage.

AVOID / WATCH OUT FOR

- Prescription drugs that can affect taste.

Arrhythmia
(Irregular Heartbeat)

Any change in the rhythm of the heartbeat is known as an arrhythmia. In general, most arrhythmias pose little or no threat besides heightened anxiety; however, when an arrhythmia is accompanied by dizziness and fainting, an immediate trip to the doctor is warranted. While there are medications one can take to regulate the heartbeat, arrhythmia without a serious underlying cause can be treated quite successfully with natural remedies.

ARRHYTHMIA (IRREGULAR HEARTBEAT)

SUPPLEMENTS

- Calcium: 1,000 mg daily (older women: 1,500–2,000 mg).
- Coenzyme Q_{10}: 120 mg daily.
- Complete all-natural multivitamin/mineral complex rich in antioxidants.
- Magnesium: 500 mg daily.
- Vitamin E complex (with tocotrienols): 400–800 IU daily.

HERBS

- Garlic extract: 500–1,000 mg daily.
- Grape seed extract: 200 mg daily.
- Green tea extract: 200 mg daily.
- Hawthorne extract: 600 mg daily.

CONSIDER / TRY TO

- Eat more fish rich in omega-3 fatty acids, such as salmon, mackerel, herring, tuna and cod, twice weekly.
- Exercise regularly.
- Lose weight.
- Reduce stress using biofeedback, acupuncture, breathing exercises, or just listening to good music.

AVOID / WATCH OUT FOR

- Alcohol.
- Caffeine.
- Smoking.
- Margarine and hydrogenated or partially hydrogenated vegetable oils (trans fatty acids).

Arthritis

Arthritis is the inflammation of a joint or joints, usually accompanied by pain, restricted motion, warmth, and swelling. There are more than 200 causes of arthritis; rheumatoid arthritis and osteoarthritis are the most well known. Rheumatoid arthritis is an autoimmune disease that can affect anyone at any stage of life, while osteoarthritis is a degenerative disorder that is usually associated with advanced age. Certain nutritional supplements and herbs can help reduce joint inflammation, thereby easing the associated pain.

ARTHRITIS

SUPPLEMENTS

- Bioflavonoids: 500 mg daily.
- Chondroitin sulfate: 1,000–2,000 mg daily.
- Digestive enzymes: one to three capsules with each meal.
- Glucosamine sulfate potassium: 700–1,050 mg daily.
- Omega-3 fatty acids (fish oil capsules): 50 mg, one to three times daily.

HERBS

- Cat's claw: as directed on label.
- Feverfew: as directed on label.
- Ginger extract (EV EXT 77): 170 mg, one to three times daily (as capsules).
- Ginseng: as directed on label.
- Licorice root: 450 mg, one to three times daily (as capsules).
- White willow bark: as directed on label.

CONSIDER / TRY TO

- Acupressure.
- Detoxification (see TOXICITY on page 280).
- Exercise moderately.
- Yoga.

AVOID / WATCH OUT FOR

- Environmental toxins, including pesticides.
- Food allergies.
- Hydrogenated oils.
- Junk food and fatty, greasy foods.
- NSAIDs (nonsteroidal anti-inflammatory drugs), such as aspirin and ibuprofen.

27

Asthma

In asthma, there is a widespread narrowing of the bronchial airways, which leads to coughing, wheezing, and difficulty breathing. In susceptible individuals, asthmatic reactions can be triggered by certain stimuli, such as exercise, cold air, and allergens, including pollen, animal dander, and dust mites. Stress and anxiety can also trigger an asthma attack. In some cases, this condition can be life threatening and should be treated accordingly. Natural remedies for asthma can help reduce the severity and frequency of attacks.

SUPPLEMENTS

- Magnesium: 250–500 mg daily.
- Multi–trace mineral formula: as directed on label.
- Vitamin B complex: 25–50 mg daily.
- Vitamin C: 500–1,000 mg with 500 mg of bioflavonoids daily.

HERBS

- Ginger extract (EV EXT 77): 170 mg, one to two times daily (as capsules).
- Ginseng: as directed on label.
- Licorice root: 450 mg, one to three times daily (as capsules).

CONSIDER / TRY TO

- Acupuncture.
- Detoxification (see TOXICITY on page 280).
- Immune-system boosters (see IMMUNE SYSTEM, WEAKENED on page 164).
- Meditation and/or yoga.
- Use dust mite protectors and an air purifier in your home.

AVOID / WATCH OUT FOR

- Allergies to dust, pollen, mold, and dander.
- Leaky gut syndrome.
- Stress.
- Synthetic estrogens/progestins (birth control pills and HRT).

Atherosclerosis

Atherosclerosis is a condition in which an artery or arteries become clogged with deposits of fatty material, mainly cholesterol. Depending on which arteries are affected, atherosclerosis can lead to stroke, heart attack, or other complications. Symptoms, such as pain in the legs and chest, usually do not occur until the disease is well advanced. Therefore, if you have known risk factors for atherosclerosis, which include, among others, high blood pressure, high cholesterol, and diabetes, it is especially important to take the natural steps suggested here to avoid or curtail its progression.

ATHEROSCLEROSIS

SUPPLEMENTS

- Alpha lipoic acid: 50 mg daily.
- Calcium: 1,000 mg daily (older women: 1,500–2,000 mg).
- Coenzyme Q_{10}: 120 mg daily.
- Folic acid: 400 mcg daily.
- L-Arginine: 1,000 mg, two to three times daily.
- Magnesium: 500 mg daily.
- Vitamin E complex (with tocotrienols): 400–800 IU daily.

HERBS

- Capsicum extract: 10 mg daily.
- Garlic extract: 500–1,000 mg daily.
- Grape seed: 200 mg daily.
- Green tea extract: 200 mg daily.
- Hawthorne extract: 600 mg daily.

CONSIDER / TRY TO

- Drink eight to ten glasses of pure water daily.
- Eat generous amounts of fresh garlic and onions.
- Increase your consumption of whole foods, such as fresh fruits and vegetables, nuts, seeds, legumes, fish, and beans.
- Reduce stress.
- Weight-loss diet.

AVOID / WATCH OUT FOR

- Processed foods, especially sugar, white flour, and other refined carbohydrates.
- Trans fatty acids, such as margarine, hydrogenated and partially hydrogenated oils.

Athlete's Foot

Athlete's foot, also known as foot ringworm, is a common skin infection caused by fungi that thrive in the warm, moist areas between the toes. Symptoms can range from mild scaling to an itchy, painful rash, and in more severe cases, fluid-filled blisters. The infection can spread from the toes to the bottoms and sides of the feet. In addition to natural remedies, keeping the feet clean and dry and wearing shoes that allow the feet to breathe work well to clear up the infection and keep the risk of reinfection minimal. See also FUNGAL SKIN INFECTIONS.

SUPPLEMENTS

- MSM: 1,000 mg, one to three times daily.
- Probiotics: one to three capsules *or* one tablespoon of refrigerated liquid probiotics, one to three times daily before meals; *or* acidophilus: one to three (multi-billion count) capsules before meals.
- Vitamin B complex: 25–50 mg daily.
- Vitamin C: 500–1,000 mg daily.
- Zinc: 15 mg of elemental zinc (read label), once or twice daily.

HERBS

- Garlic: 500 mg daily.
- Tea tree oil: apply topically twice daily.

CONSIDER / TRY TO

- Keep feet dry.
- Soak feet in mixture of vinegar and water.

AVOID / WATCH OUT FOR

- Bare feet in public locker rooms.
- Fried, greasy foods.
- Processed foods.
- Sugar and sugary beverages.

Backaches/Back Pain

Aches and pains in the back can be symptoms of any number of conditions, including muscle strain, injury, osteoarthritis, and pregnancy. Steps should be taken to determine the cause of the pain. If the cause of the pain is due to strain, injury, or overuse, resting, supplementing with nutrients and herbs, and trying alternative healthcare treatments, such as chiropractic, all can provide relief. Activities, such as lifting heavy boxes, should be avoided whenever possible; if necessary, however, proper lifting techniques can reduce the risk of injury or strain.

SUPPLEMENTS

- Calcium: 500–1,000 mg daily (older women: 1,500–2,000 mg).
- DLPA (dl-phenylalanine): 375–750 mg, every four hours for discomfort (as capsules).
- Glucosamine sulfate potassium: 700–1,050 mg daily.
- Magnesium: 250–500 mg daily.
- Multi–trace mineral formula: as directed on label.

HERBS

- Feverfew: as directed on label.
- St. John's wort (dual action): 300 mg, once or twice daily.
- White willow bark: 500–1,000 mg, two to three times daily (as capsules).

CONSIDER / TRY TO

- Acupuncture.
- Chiropractic.
- Exercises for back and stomach muscles.
- Lose excess weight.
- Yoga.

AVOID / WATCH OUT FOR

- Constipation.
- Extra body weight.
- High heels.
- Improper lifting.
- Overdoing exercise.

Bad Breath (Halitosis)

Bad breath (halitosis) can be either a temporary or a chronic condition. Temporary bad breath can result from eating certain foods, such as onions or garlic; smoking; or taking certain prescription drugs. Chronic bad breath can have more serious causes, including tooth or gum disease, poor digestion, liver disease, and diabetes. Frequent proper brushing, including a light brushing of the tongue, and flossing are, of course, the first line of treatment. Nutritional supplements and other steps can be taken to reduce or eliminate unpleasant odor.

BAD BREATH (HALITOSIS)

SUPPLEMENTS

- Acidophilus: one to three (multi-billion count) capsules before each meal.
- Betaine hydrochloride (HCL): 150 mg with each meal (as capsules).
- Digestive enzymes: one to three capsules with each meal.
- Vitamin A: 5,000–10,000 IU daily.
- Vitamin B complex: 25–50 mg daily.
- Vitamin C: 500–1,000 mg daily.
- Zinc: 15 mg of elemental zinc (read label), once or twice daily.

HERBS

- Chlorophyll: as directed on label.
- Parsley: as directed on label.

CONSIDER / TRY TO

- Detoxification (see TOXICITY on page 280).
- Drink six to eight glasses of pure water daily.
- Eat more fiber-rich foods.
- Eat more raw fruits and vegetables.
- Use dental floss.

AVOID / WATCH OUT FOR

- Mouthwash containing sugar, alcohol, and dyes.
- Offending foods.

Bad Breath (Halitosis)

Bedsores

Bedsores (or skin ulcers) commonly develop in people with limited movement who are confined to beds or wheelchairs. Ulcers develop when constant pressure prevents or interrupts oxygen-rich blood from getting to all layers of the skin. Without oxygen, the skin dies, layer by layer. Without intervention, deep sores and infection may result. Bedsores can be prevented by changing positions often and heal more quickly with natural remedies.

SUPPLEMENTS

- Complete all-natural multivitamin/mineral complex rich in antioxidants.
- Glutamine: 50–150 mg daily in divided dosage.
- MSM lotion: apply topically up to three times daily.
- MSM (with vitamin C complex): 1,000 mg, three times daily.
- Vitamin C complex: 500–1,000 mg daily.
- Zinc: 15 mg of elemental zinc, once or twice daily.

HERBS

- Comfrey, calendula, and aloe vera topical ointment: apply topically up to three times daily.

CONSIDER / TRY TO

- Change sleeping positions frequently.
- Keep sheets clean, dry, and tight.
- Keep skin clean and dry.
- Massage the affected areas of the skin.

AVOID / WATCH OUT FOR

- Alcohol.
- Caffeine.
- Processed foods, especially sugar, white flour, and other refined carbohydrates.
- Smoking or breathing secondhand smoke.
- Tight-fitting clothes.

Bedwetting

It is not uncommon for preadolescent children to wet the bed once in a while; this is no cause for concern. However, frequent bed-wetting does require parental and sometimes medical intervention. Although rarely a cause, a urinary tract infection could be the culprit and should be ruled out. It is important to remember that the bed-wetting is accidental and should not be a cause for punishment. Many children outgrow bed-wetting on their own, but there are steps you can take to help your child overcome the problem naturally.

SUPPLEMENTS

- All-natural children's multivitamin/mineral.
- Calcium: 100 mg daily.
- Magnesium: 25 mg daily.
- Potassium: 25 mg daily.

HERBS

- St. John's wort (children's dosage dual action): 150 mg, once daily at bedtime (ages six to twelve; children under age six should seek professional help).

CONSIDER / TRY TO

- Leave a dim light on in the bedroom to encourage getting up at night to use the bathroom.

AVOID / WATCH OUT FOR

- Any liquids one hour before bedtime.
- Caffeine.
- Diabetes.
- Food and environmental allergies.
- Heavy sleeping.
- Nutritional deficiencies (namely magnesium).
- Stress.

Bell's Palsy

Bell's palsy is a condition in which the nerve on one side of the face becomes paralyzed or excessively week, causing facial distortion. Still under investigation, the cause is most likely due to swelling of the facial nerve brought on by some unknown factor(s). Most cases of Bell's palsy are temporary, and full control of the facial muscles is restored within a few months. There are no standard conventional treatments for this condition, but natural remedies can quicken recovery.

SUPPLEMENTS

- Alpha lipoic acid: 50 mg daily.
- Complete all-natural multivitamin/mineral complex rich in antioxidants.
- Evening primrose oil: 500 mg, three times daily.
- MSM (with vitamin C complex): 1,000 mg, three times daily.

HERBS

- Garlic extract: 500 mg, twice daily.
- Ginger extract (EV EXT 77): 170 mg, one to three times daily.
- Ginkgo biloba: 60 mg, twice daily.

CONSIDER / TRY TO

- Eat fish such as salmon, mackerel, herring, tuna, and cod, twice weekly.
- Eat one pint of plain, unsweetened live-cultured yogurt daily to promote proper digestion.

AVOID / WATCH OUT FOR

- Alcohol and other recreational drugs.
- Caffeine.
- Foods containing artificial flavorings, colors, preservatives, salicylates, nitrates, nitrites, phosphates and monosodium glutamate (MSG).
- Ice cold drinks and foods such as ice cream.
- Processed foods, especially sugar, white flour, and other refined carbohydrates.
- Smoking or breathing secondhand smoke.

Bipolar Disorder

Also known as manic-depressive disorder, bipolar disorder is a chronic condition in which a person experiences mild or extreme mood swings, from episodes of depression to sudden mania (excessive excitement). Although the cause is unknown, it is generally believed that this disorder runs in families. Medication, such as a mood stabilizer, is often prescribed to even out the mood swings, and counseling and support groups often help. Additionally, following a proper diet, along with a good supplement regimen, can bring about lasting positive changes in an affected person's behavior.

SUPPLEMENTS

- L-Tyrosine: 3,000 mg daily at bedtime on an empty stomach.
- MSM (with vitamin C complex): 1,000 mg, twice daily.
- Vitamin B complex: 50 mg, twice daily with food.

HERBS

- Ginkgo biloba: 60 mg, twice daily.
- Grape seed extract: 200 mg daily.
- Green tea extract: 200 mg daily.
- St. John's wort (dual action): 300 mg, two to three times daily.

CONSIDER / TRY TO

- Eat foods rich in tryptophan, such as turkey, avocado, walnuts, bananas, dates, figs, kiwi, fruit, brown rice, and legumes.
- Increase consumption of raw, whole foods, such as fresh fruits and vegetables.
- Reduce stress.
- Spend more time outdoors.

AVOID / WATCH OUT FOR

- Foods containing artificial flavorings, colors, preservatives, salicylates, nitrates, nitrites, phosphates and monosodium glutamate (MSG).

Blood Pressure, High

The force that blood puts on the walls of the veins, arteries, and heart is known as blood pressure. High blood pressure, also called hypertension, is a condition in which the pressure is abnormally high. The cause of hypertension is unclear, and the condition can remain symptomless for years, increasing the risk of life-threatening conditions, such as heart attack, heart failure, and stroke. With proper care, including natural remedies, this condition can be controlled to prevent complications.

SUPPLEMENTS

- Coenzyme Q_{10}: 60 mg, one to three times daily.
- Magnesium: 250–500 mg daily.
- Vitamin E: 400–500 IU daily.

HERBS

- Garlic: 500 mg daily.
- Ginseng: as directed on label.
- Hawthorne extract: as directed on label.

CONSIDER / TRY TO

- Eat six stalks of celery or the juice equivalent daily.
- Exercise regularly.
- Lose weight if necessary.
- Meditation and/or yoga.
- Reduce stress.

AVOID / WATCH OUT FOR

- Chronic stress.
- High-fat diet.
- Long-term supplementation of licorice with glycyrrhizin.
- Obesity.

Blood Sugar, High/Low

Blood sugar is the amount of glucose (a simple sugar) in the blood. It is normal for blood-sugar levels to vary throughout the day. However, levels that are chronically either too high or too low indicate an underlying condition, such as diabetes or hypoglycemia, respectively. Treating the underlying condition is paramount, but steps can be taken to stabilize blood sugar naturally.

BLOOD SUGAR, HIGH/LOW

SUPPLEMENTS

- Chromium: 200–600 mg daily.
- Essential fatty acids: 250 mg, one to three times daily (as capsules).
- Inositol hexanicotinate (no-flush niacin): 250–500 mg daily.
- MSM: 1,000 mg, one to three times daily.
- Vanadium (Vanadyl): 10 mg daily.
- Vitamin C: 500–1,000 mg daily.
- Vitamin E: 400–500 IU daily.

HERBS

- Ginkgo biloba extract: 60 mg, one to three times daily.
- Ginseng: as directed on label.
- Grape seed extract (PCOs): 100 mg, one to three times daily.

CONSIDER / TRY TO

- Eat more vegetables.
- Exercise.
- Lose weight if necessary.

AVOID / WATCH OUT FOR

- All sugars and refined carbohydrates.
- Excess carbohydrates.
- Processed foods.

Breast Cancer

Breast cancer is cancer of the breast tissue.
It is classified by the type of tissue in which it
originates, such as the milk ducts or connective
tissue, and by how much it has spread.
Symptoms that may indicate breast cancer
include a lump in the breast, chronic swelling
of the breast, and changes in shape of the
breast or nipple. Treatment may involve surgery,
chemotherapy, radiation therapy, and/or
hormone-blocking drugs. Natural remedies
may help delay or avoid the onset of breast
cancer. See also CANCER PREVENTION.

SUPPLEMENTS

- Flaxseed oil (refrigerated): one teaspoon of the oil; *or* 500 mg, one to three times daily (as capsules).
- Limonene: 5–50 mg daily.
- Melatonin: 1–3 mg, just before bedtime.
- Selenium: 100–200 mcg daily.
- Soy isoflavonoids: 40–60 mg daily.

HERBS

- Psyllium: as directed on label.

CONSIDER / TRY TO

- Drink soymilk and soy shakes.
- Eat soybeans.
- Eat wheat bran.

AVOID / WATCH OUT FOR

- High-fat foods.
- Low-fiber foods.
- Processed foods.

Bronchitis

Bronchitis is an inflammation of the bronchi, or airways. It initially presents itself as a dry cough but leads to the expectoration of yellowish-green sputum within a few days. It may be accompanied by cold symptoms, such as aches and pains or a runny nose. Bronchitis is usually caused by a viral or bacterial infection, but can also result from inhaled irritants. Left untreated, severe bronchitis can lead to pneumonia, so it's important to take steps to heal the condition in its early stages. Fortunately, there are many natural ways to accomplish this.

SUPPLEMENTS

- Coenzyme Q_{10}: 50 mg, twice daily.
- Complete all-natural multivitamin/mineral complex rich in antioxidants.
- Glutamine: 50–150 mg, divided doses daily.
- Omega-3 fatty acids: 1,000 mg daily (as fish oil capsules).
- Quercetin: 500 mg, twice daily.

HERBS

- Astragalus: 200 mg, three times daily.
- Ginkgo biloba: 60 mg, twice daily.
- Grape seed extract: 200 mg daily.
- Green tea extract: 200 mg daily.
- Licorice root tea: one cup daily.

CONSIDER / TRY TO

- Eat a high-protein diet, including fish, lean meats free of hormones and antibiotics, and free range poultry.
- Increase consumption of fresh fruits and vegetables.
- Use a heating pad on your chest and back at night.

AVOID / WATCH OUT FOR

- Air pollution.
- Cough suppressants.
- Dairy products and refined carbohydrates.
- Smoking.

Bruises

Bruises form from breakages of small blood vessels in the skin. Blood leaks out of the damaged vessels, leaving red dots or bluish-purple marks that fade over time. It is normal for bruises to develop from a hard blow to the body; however, chronic bruising may indicate a problem with blood-clotting. Such a problem can be determined through blood tests. Bruises respond very well to natural therapies. Nutritional supplements and herbs applied topically can speed recovery time and help the bruise fade quickly.

SUPPLEMENTS

- Coenzyme Q_{10}: 60 mg, one to three times daily.
- Digestive enzymes: one to three capsules with each meal.
- Rutin: 50 mg, one to three times daily.
- Vitamin A: 5,000–10,000 IU daily.
- Vitamin C: 500–1,000 mg with 500 mg of bioflavonoids daily.
- Vitamin E: 400–500 IU daily.

HERBS

- Aloe vera gel: apply topically as directed on label.
- Arnica homeopathic tablets: dissolve under tongue as directed on label.
- Calendula ointment or gel: apply topically as directed on label.
- Comfrey: apply topically as directed on label.
- Garlic: 500 mg daily.
- White willow bark: 500–1,000 mg, two to three times daily (as capsules).
- Witch hazel: apply topical preparation as directed on label.

CONSIDER / TRY TO

- Apply an ice pack.
- Eat leafy green vegetables and fresh fruit, especially pineapple.
- Homeopathic bruise remedy.

AVOID / WATCH OUT FOR

- Taking aspirin in excess (more than six 325-mg tablets per day).

Bruxism (Teeth Grinding)

To some extent, we all grind our teeth, but some people do it excessively—albeit unconsciously. There are several theories as to why this occurs, but no one particular cause has been pinpointed. In susceptible individuals, bruxism often occurs during times of stress or while asleep. This constant grinding results in the wearing away of the tooth's enamel and causes pain in the jaw. Conventional treatment ranges from relaxation techniques to mouth guards, but other steps, including a good supplement regimen, can help.

BRUXISM (TEETH GRINDING)

SUPPLEMENTS

- Calcium: 1,000 mg daily (older women: 1,500–2,000 mg).
- Complete all-natural multivitamin/mineral complex rich in antioxidants.
- Magnesium: 500 mg daily.

HERBS

- Omega-3 fatty acids: 1,000 mg daily (as fish oil capsules).
- Passion flower and hops tea natural calming agents: daily.
- St. John's wort (dual action): 300 mg, two to three times daily.
- Valerian extract: 2–3 grams at bedtime.

CONSIDER / TRY TO

- Bite alignment from your dentist.
- Eat a high-protein diet.
- Eat foods rich in omega-3 fatty acids, such as salmon, tuna, herring, and cod, twice weekly.
- Exercise regularly.
- Increase consumption of raw whole foods.
- Reduce stress.

AVOID / WATCH OUT FOR

- Caffeine.
- Foods containing artificial flavorings, colors, preservatives, salicylates, nitrates, nitrites, phosphates and monosodium glutamate (MSG).
- Processed foods, especially sugar, white flour, and other refined carbohydrates.
- Smoking or breathing secondhand smoke.

Burns

Burns occur when the skin is exposed to high heat, certain chemicals, or intense electrical currents. Sometimes the underlying tissue and, in severe cases, the internal organs can be damaged. Burns range from first degree (the least severe) to third degree (the most severe). Minor burns respond well to home treatment; however, severe burns require immediate medical care. For minor burns and recovery from severe burns, natural remedies can provide much-needed relief and quicker healing.

SUPPLEMENTS

- Coenzyme Q_{10}: 60 mg, one to three times daily.
- MSM: 1,000 mg, one to three times daily.
- Potassium: 99 mg, one to three times daily.
- Selenium: 100–200 mcg daily.
- Vitamin A: 5,000–10,000 IU daily.
- Vitamin C: 500–1,000 mg daily.
- Vitamin E: 400–500 IU daily.
- Zinc: 15 mg of elemental zinc (read label), once or twice daily.

HERBS

- Aloe vera gel: apply topically as directed on label.

CONSIDER / TRY TO

- Apply a cold compress to the burn.
- Drink eight to ten glasses of pure water daily.
- High-protein diet.
- Homeopathic burn remedy.
- Use a bacteria-killing spray.

AVOID / WATCH OUT FOR

- Do not apply any type of butter to the burn.
- Do not break blisters.

Cancer Prevention

Cancer is one of the most dreaded diseases. It results from abnormal, uncontrollable cell growth and can affect any tissue in the body. That's why there are so many different types of cancer. Both genetic and environmental factors can increase the risk of developing this often life-threatening disease. If you are at high risk, it would serve you well to follow a cancer-preventive daily regimen, including nutritional supplements and healthy foods, and to avoid cancer-causing substances, such as cigarette smoke and environmental toxins. See also BREAST CANCER; CERVICAL CANCER; COLON CANCER; LUNG CANCER; ORAL CANCER; PROSTATE CANCER; RECTAL CANCER; SKIN CANCER; STOMACH CANCER.

SUPPLEMENTS

- Cysteine: 100–250 mg, one to two times daily.
- Folic acid: 400–800 mcg daily.
- Glutathione: 50 mg, one to three times daily.
- Manganese: 9 mg daily.
- Selenium: 100–200 mcg daily.
- Vitamin A: 5,000–10,000 IU daily.
- Vitamin B_6 (pyridoxine): 25–50 mg daily.
- Vitamin E: 400–500 IU daily.
- Zinc: 15 mg of elemental zinc (read label), once or twice daily.

HERBS

- Cat's claw: as directed on label.
- Garlic: 500 mg daily.
- Ginseng: as directed on label.
- Quercetin: 400 mg before eating, one to three times daily.

CONSIDER / TRY TO

- Detoxification (see TOXICITY on page 280).
- Eat legumes/beans and soy products.
- Eat more fiber-rich foods.
- Eat more red, yellow, and orange fruits and vegetables.

AVOID / WATCH OUT FOR

- Emotional stress.
- Environmental toxins, such as pesticides and herbicides.
- Food additives.
- Radiation.
- Smoking.

Candidiasis

Candidiasis is a yeastlike fungal infection of the muscous membranes caused by the various strains of *Candida,* most usually *C. albicans.* Symptoms, such as white patches in the mouth or red skin lesions, vary depending on the infection site. Common sites include the mouth, vagina, respiratory tract, and the skin folds. In rare cases, it may spread throughout the body. Usually treated with antifungal drugs, this condition responds well to natural remedies. See also FUNGAL SKIN INFECTIONS; VAGINAL YEAST INFECTION.

SUPPLEMENTS

- Digestive enzymes: one to three capsules with each meal.
- Essential fatty acids: 250 mg, one to three times daily (as capsules).
- MSM: 1,000 mg, one to three times daily.
- Complete all-natural multivitamin/mineral complex rich in antioxidants.
- Probiotics: one to three capsules *or* one tablespoon of refrigerated liquid probiotics, up to three times daily before meals; or acidophilus: one to three (multi-billion count) capsules before meals.
- Selenium: 100–200 mcg daily.

HERBS

- Garlic: 500 mg daily.

CONSIDER / TRY TO

- Cleansing diet.
- Detoxification (see TOXICITY on page 280).
- Vinegar or yogurt douche.

AVOID / WATCH OUT FOR

- Alcohol, sugar, and yeast.
- Antibiotics and oral contraceptives.
- Chemical cleaners.
- Highly alkaline and acid foods.
- Mold.
- Mothballs.

Canker Sores

Canker sores are painful, benign ulcerations of the lips and/or mouth. The exact cause of these annoying sores remains unknown, and indeed several factors probably play a role, including nutritional deficiencies and a weakened immune system. The sores should heal on their own within a few days to a couple of weeks, but in the meantime, the discomfort may seem unbearable. Natural pain-relieving remedies and immune boosters can make the pain less intense while helping to speed along the healing process.

SUPPLEMENTS

- Glutamine: 50–150 mg daily.
- L-Lysine: 500 mg, three times daily between meals.
- MSM (with vitamin C complex): as directed on label.

HERBS

- Echinacea: 100–500 mg daily for two weeks.
- Garlic extract: 500 mg, twice daily.
- Grape seed extract: 200 mg daily.
- Green tea extract: 200 mg daily.
- Omega-3 fatty acids: 1,000 mg daily (as fish oil capsules).

CONSIDER / TRY TO

- Apply ice cube to canker sore to reduce pain and inflammation.
- Eat foods rich in omega-3 fatty acids, such as salmon, tuna, herring, and cod, twice weekly.
- Increase consumption of whole foods, fresh vegetables, and fruits.
- Rinse your mouth several times daily with a mixture of warm water and half a teaspoon of salt.
- Use all-natural organic toothpaste and mouthwash.
- Use soft toothbrush and floss after each meal.

AVOID / WATCH OUT FOR

- Alcohol.
- Caffeine.
- Chewing gum.
- Extremely hot foods.
- Hydrogenated, partially hydrogenated, or trans fatty acid oils.
- Spicy and highly acidic food.
- Stress.
- Sugar and refined carbohydrates.

Cardiomyopathy

A life-threatening condition, cardiomyopathy is any disorder of the heart muscle—specifically, the muscular walls of the ventricles, or the lower chambers of the heart. There are several types of cardiomyopathy, including dilated cardiomyopathy, hypertrophic cardiomyopathy, and restrictive cardiomyopathy, as well as several causes, including heart disease, alcohol or drug abuse, and genetics. While muscle damage usually cannot be reversed, natural steps can be taken along with conventional treatment to improve overall health and longevity.

SUPPLEMENTS

- Calcium: 1,000 mg daily (older women: 1,500–2,000 mg).
- Coenzyme Q_{10}: 60 mg, one to three times daily (as capsules).
- Complete all-natural multivitamin/mineral complex rich in antioxidants.
- L-Arginine: 1,500 mg, twice daily (as timed-release capsule).
- Magnesium: 500 mg daily.
- Vitamin E complex (with tocotrienols): 400–800 IU daily.

HERBS

- Capsicum extract: 10 mg daily.
- Grape seed extract: 200 mg daily.
- Green tea extract: 200 mg daily.
- Hawthorne extract: 600 mg daily.
- Omega-3 fatty acids: 1,000 mg daily (as fish oil capsules).

CONSIDER / TRY TO

- Eat foods rich in omega-3 fatty acids, such as salmon, tuna, herring, and cod, twice weekly.
- Exercise regularly.
- Increase consumption of whole foods, fresh vegetables, and fruits.
- Quit smoking.
- Reduce stress.

AVOID / WATCH OUT FOR

- Alcohol.
- Caffeine.
- Hydrogenated vegetable oils and trans fatty acids.
- Pesticides, solvents, and all other environmental toxins.

Cardiovascular Disease

Cardiovascular disease is a catchall term for disorders of the heart and blood vessels, including heart attack, stroke, and heart failure. A properly functioning cardiovascular system is essential for the circulation of blood around the body. A block in the flow of blood anywhere in the body can have devastating effects. Therefore, preventing and controlling this disease is extremely important. There are many natural steps a person can take to manage an existing cardiovascular condition, including taking supplements and making important lifestyle changes. See also STROKE.

SUPPLEMENTS

- Coenzyme Q_{10}: 60 mg, one to three times daily.
- Cysteine: 100–250 mg, one to two times daily.
- Glutathione: 50 mg, one to three times daily.
- Magnesium: 250–500 mg daily.
- Selenium: 100–200 mcg daily.
- Vitamin B complex: 25–50 mg daily.
- Vitamin C: 500–1,000 mg daily.
- Vitamin E: 400–500 IU daily.

HERBS

- Cayenne: as directed on label.
- Garlic: 500 mg daily.
- Ginseng: as directed on label.
- Hawthorne extract: as directed on label.

CONSIDER / TRY TO

- Drink red wine in moderation.
- Eat high-fiber foods and soy products.
- Eat less red meat and more fish.
- Eat more vegetables and fruit.
- Exercise regularly.
- Lose weight if necessary.
- Reduce dietary fat.

AVOID / WATCH OUT FOR

- Processed foods.
- Refined and hydrogenated oils.
- Salt and sugar.
- Smoking.
- Stress.
- Too much coffee and tea (more than three cups daily).

Carpal Tunnel Syndrome

CARPAL TUNNEL SYNDROME

Carpal tunnel syndrome is a relatively common condition of one or both hands resulting from compression of the nerve that travels through the wrist. Repetitive movements of the hands, such as typing or using a screwdriver, have been implicated as a cause. Symptoms include numbness, tingling, and pain, sometimes traveling up to the arms and shoulders. Avoiding aggravating positions, along with taking nutritional supplements, can often provide relief.

SUPPLEMENTS

- MSM: 1,000 mg, one to three times daily.
- Vitamin B complex: 25–50 mg daily.
- Vitamin B_6 (pyridoxine): 25–50 mg daily.

HERBS

- Ginger extract (EV EXT 77): one capsule, three times daily with food.

CONSIDER / TRY TO

- Stretch the hands, wrists, arms, and shoulders every fifteen minutes.
- Massage.
- Move keyboard to a different position.
- Slope chair slightly forward.

AVOID / WATCH OUT FOR

- Repetitive motions.
- Sitting in same position for long periods.

Cataracts

A cataract is an opacity, or clouding, of the eye's lens. The clouding results in blurred vision, which progressively worsens, leading to blindness. This condition is most commonly seen in people of advanced age, but may occur earlier in its congenital form or as a complication of other diseases, such as diabetes. A cataract will not improve on its own, and surgery may become necessary to restore sight. However, the progression may be slowed by taking nutritional supplements and by following some commonsense advice. See also VISION PROBLEMS.

SUPPLEMENTS

- Beta-carotene: 10,000–20,000 IU daily.
- Complete all-natural multivitamin/mineral complex rich in antioxidants.
- Glutathione: 50 mg, one to three times daily.
- Lutein: 6–20 mg daily.
- Quercetin: 400 mg before eating, one to three times daily.
- Riboflavin (vitamin B_2): 50–100 mg daily.
- Vitamin C: 500–1,000 mg daily.
- Vitamin E: 400–500 IU daily.
- Zeaxanthin: 30–130 mg daily.

HERBS

- Bilberry extract: as directed on label.
- Marigold: as directed on label.

CONSIDER / TRY TO

- Eat more fresh fruits and vegetables.
- Wear good quality sunglasses with UV-ray protection.

AVOID / WATCH OUT FOR

- Direct exposure to sunlight for long periods.
- Smoking.

Cavities (Tooth Decay)

Dental caries, commonly called cavities, are caused by acid-producing bacteria that slowly eat away at the tooth's enamel. Once through the enamel, they rapidly work their way toward the innermost part of the tooth, known as the pulp. Deep cavities may require root canal and even extraction of the tooth. Besides the obvious—avoiding sugary foods, brushing and flossing regularly, and getting regular cleanings—there are many steps you can take to reduce the chance that this unwanted bacteria will wreak havoc in your mouth.

CAVITIES (TOOTH DECAY)

SUPPLEMENTS

- Calcium: 1,000 mg daily (older women: 1,500–2,000 mg).
- Complete all-natural multivitamin/mineral complex rich in antioxidants.
- Magnesium: 500 mg daily.
- MSM (with vitamin C complex): 1,000 mg, twice daily.

HERBS

- Grape seed extract: 200 mg daily.

CONSIDER / TRY TO

- Apply aloe vera gel and clove oil to inflamed gums.
- Drink several cups of green tea daily.
- Reduce stress.

AVOID / WATCH OUT FOR

- Alcohol.
- Mercury fillings.
- Processed foods, especially sugar, white flour, and other refined carbohydrates.
- Smoking.
- Teeth grinding.

Cervical Cancer

Cancer of the cervix—the outer edge of the uterus—is one of the more common cancers of the female reproductive system. Women between the ages of thirty-five and fifty-five are most often affected. Often symptomless until the late stages of the disease, cervical cancer usually can be detected by a Pap test. Taking nutritional supplements and making simple lifestyle changes can reduce the risk of this type of cancer, and can only benefit those who have it. See also CANCER PREVENTION.

SUPPLEMENTS

- Folic acid: 400–800 mcg daily.
- Lycopene: 6–10 mg daily.
- Vitamin B_{12}: 100–1,000 mcg daily.

HERBS

- No herbs apply.

CONSIDER / TRY TO

- Eat more tomatoes, citrus fruits, whole grains, yeast, liver, and dark green vegetables.

AVOID / WATCH OUT FOR

- Multiple sex partners.
- Smoking.

Chickenpox

Characterized by itchy red spots, chickenpox is
a highly contagious infection with the varicella-
zoster virus. Although it is commonly thought of
as a childhood condition, it can occur in anyone
of any age, and is actually more serious when
it affects older individuals. Moreover, after the
initial infection, the virus remains dormant in
the body, and may present itself as shingles
years later. In general, chickenpox clears up
within a few weeks, but the use of natural
remedies can speed the process along as
well as relieve the associated discomfort.

SUPPLEMENTS

- Children's multivitamin/mineral.
- MSM: 1,000 mg, two to three times daily.
- Zinc: 15 mg of elemental zinc, once or twice daily.

HERBS

- Astragalus: 200 mg, twice daily.
- Elderberry extract: one teaspoon, twice daily.
- Olive leaf extract: 250 mg, twice daily.

CONSIDER / TRY TO

- Keep chicken pox clean and dry to prevent secondary infections.
- Warm baths with cornstarch or oatmeal (uncooked) sprinkled in to help relieve excessive itching.
- Wear loose-fitting clothing.

AVOID / WATCH OUT FOR

- Aspirin.
- Dairy products.
- Foods rich in trans fatty acids.
- Over-exposing areas of the skin affected by chicken pox to direct sunlight for more than fifteen minutes per day.
- Scratching.
- Smoking or breathing secondhand smoke.

Cholesterol, Elevated

Cholesterol is one of the two major fats found in the blood. While the body needs this fat to perform certain functions, too much of the "bad" type (LDL cholesterol) circulating in the bloodstream can contribute to problems such as heart disease. Several factors can increase cholesterol levels, including diabetes, a diet high in saturated fats, and heredity. Fortunately, elevated cholesterol levels respond well to nutritional supplements and moderate lifestyle changes.

SUPPLEMENTS

- Calcium: 500–1,000 mg daily (older women: 1,500–2,000 mg).
- Coenzyme Q_{10}: 60 mg, one to three times daily.
- Glutathione: 50 mg, one to three times daily.
- Inositol hexanicotinate (no-flush niacin): 250–500 mg daily.
- L-Carnitine: 50–500 mg daily.
- Magnesium: 250–500 mg daily.
- Policosanol: 10 mg daily.
- Vitamin A: 5,000–10,000 IU daily.
- Vitamin C: 500–1,000 mg daily.
- Vitamin D: 200–800 IU daily.
- Vitamin E: 400–500 IU daily.
- Vitamin K: 100 mcg daily.

HERBS

- Cayenne: as directed on label.
- Garlic: 500 mg daily.
- Green tea extract: 100 mg, twice daily.

CONSIDER / TRY TO

- Eat fish, berries, olive oil, fiber-rich foods, whole grains, soy products, and yogurt.
- Exercise regularly.
- Lose weight if necessary.

AVOID / WATCH OUT FOR

- Cholesterol-lowering drugs.
- Fried foods.
- Rancid fats and hydrogenated oils.

Chronic Fatigue Syndrome (CFS)

Chronic fatigue syndrome (CFS) is a disorder characterized by extreme fatigue, low-grade fever, headaches, muscle aches, and impaired memory and/or concentration. The cause of this condition, which can last from twenty-four hours to several years, remains unknown. Care should be taken to rule out other causes of fatigue as a number of conditions may cause similar symptoms. If CFS is the problem, natural remedies can increase energy and relieve the associated aches and pains. See also FATIGUE.

CHRONIC FATIGUE SYNDROME (CFS)

SUPPLEMENTS

- Coenzyme Q_{10}: 60 mg, one to three times daily.
- DHEA: 25 mg daily for women over forty; 50 mg daily for men over forty.
- L-Carnitine: 50–500 mg daily.
- Kelp: 150 mcg daily.
- Vitamin B complex: 25–50 mg daily.
- Zinc: 15 mg of elemental zinc (read label), once or twice daily.

HERBS

- Siberian ginseng: as directed on label.
- Suma: as directed on label.

CONSIDER / TRY TO

- Eat grains, poultry, fish, eggs, beans, nuts, soy products, vegetables, and fruit.
- Yoga and deep breathing exercises.

AVOID / WATCH OUT FOR

- Coffee.
- Refined carbohydrates.
- Sugar.

Circulation, Poor

Poor circulation can affect any area of the body, but people with this condition commonly complain of having cold or numb hands and/or feet. Poor circulation can be a symptom of an underlying medical condition, which should be ruled out, or it may simply be the body's reaction to extreme changes in temperature. In either case, there are several natural ways to improve the body's circulation to reduce the discomfort associated with this condition.

SUPPLEMENTS

- Calcium: 500–1,000 mg daily (older women: 1,500–2,000 mg).
- Coenzyme Q_{10}: 60 mg, one to three times daily.
- L-Carnitine: 50–500 mg daily.
- Magnesium: 250–500 mg daily.
- Omega-3 fatty acids: 50 mg, one to three times daily (as fish oil capsules).
- Vitamin B complex: 25–50 mg daily.
- Vitamin C: 500–1,000 mg daily.
- Vitamin E: 400–500 IU daily.

HERBS

- Cayenne: as directed on label.
- Ginger extract (EV EXT 77): 170 mg, one to two times daily (as capsules).
- Ginkgo biloba extract: 60 mg, one to three times daily.
- Green tea extract: 100 mg, twice daily.
- Hawthorne extract: as directed on label.

CONSIDER / TRY TO

- Drink red wine.
- Eat more fiber-rich foods.
- Eat more onions.
- Exercise regularly.
- Lose weight if necessary.
- Massage.

AVOID / WATCH OUT FOR

- Hydrogenated oils.
- Processed foods.
- Smoking.
- Sugar.

Cirrhosis

Cirrhosis is a very serious disorder in which there is irreversible scarring of the liver. This scarring interferes with the liver's ability to perform its essential functions, including filtering the blood and manufacturing nutrients. The causes of cirrhosis are varied and include chronic alcohol abuse, hepatitis, and chronic exposure to toxins. While cirrhosis can't be reversed, its progression can be slowed and aggravating factors can be eliminated with a little help from nature.

SUPPLEMENTS

- Complete all-natural multivitamin/mineral complex rich in antioxidants.
- Evening primrose oil: 500 mg daily (as capsules).
- Glutamine: 50–150 mg daily.

HERBS

- Grape seed extract: 200 mg daily.
- Green tea extract: 200 mg daily.
- Milk thistle: 200 mg, three times daily.
- Schizandra extract: as directed on label.

CONSIDER / TRY TO

- Drink eight to ten glasses of pure water daily.
- Eat organic, pesticide-free whole foods.
- Exercise regularly.

AVOID / WATCH OUT FOR

- Alcohol.
- Caffeine.
- Foods rich in trans fatty acids.
- Prescription and over-the-counter drugs unless absolutely necessary.
- Smoking and breathing secondhand smoke.

Colds and Flu

COLDS AND FLU

The common cold and the flu, or influenza, are both caused by a variety of viruses, and both are highly contagious. Symptoms of a cold include sneezing, runny nose, and watery eyes, usually without a fever. The flu, on the other hand, has several additional symptoms, including chills, fever, and sometimes nausea and vomiting. Both conditions respond well to natural remedies. In fact, during cold and flu season, natural remedies can help boost your resistance to these viruses.

SUPPLEMENTS

- Selenium: 100–200 mcg daily.
- Vitamin A: 5,000–10,000 IU daily.
- Vitamin C: 500–1,000 mg daily.
- Vitamin E: 400–500 IU daily.
- Zinc lozenges: one lozenge dissolved in mouth, two to three times daily.

HERBS

- Echinacea: as directed on label.
- Elderberry: as directed on label.
- Feverfew: as directed on label.
- Garlic: 500 mg daily.
- Ginger extract (EV EXT 77): 170 mg, one to two times daily (as capsules).
- Goldenseal: as directed on label.
- Slippery elm: as directed on label.

CONSIDER / TRY TO

- Drink hot liquids (chicken soup and teas).
- Drink more fluids.
- Facial steam with a few drops of eucalyptus oil.
- Get extra rest.
- Saltwater nasal drops.

AVOID / WATCH OUT FOR

- Overexertion.
- Stress.
- Sugar.

Cold Sores

Also known as fever blisters, cold sores are generally caused by infection with herpes simplex virus type I. (While type II generally causes genital herpes, both types can affect either region.) Although it is virtually impossible to eliminate the virus from the body, it is possible to reduce the frequency and severity of outbreaks. Antiviral medication is often prescribed for this purpose, but there are many natural self-care techniques that can be implemented with lasting success.

SUPPLEMENTS

- Glutamine: 50–150 mg daily.
- L-Lysine: 500 mg, three times daily between meals.
- MSM: 1,000 mg, three times daily.

HERBS

- Astragalus: 400 mg, twice daily.
- Echinacea: 100–500 mg daily.
- Elderberry: one teaspoon, twice daily.
- Olive leaf extract: 500 mg, twice daily.

CONSIDER / TRY TO

- Apply ice to affected areas every ten minutes for an hour.
- Apply MSM lotion to sores.
- Eat whole foods.
- Low-carbohydrate diet.
- Reduce stress.

AVOID / WATCH OUT FOR

- Alcohol.
- Avoid foods high in arginine, including chocolate, corn, nuts, grains, beans, chicken, barley, and dairy products.
- Caffeine.
- Foods rich in trans fatty acids.

Colon Cancer

Colon cancer is cancer of the large intestines. Diet, heredity, ulcerative colitis, and Crohn's disease all seem to play a part in increasing the risk of developing this disease. Once discovered, the infected segment of the intestines is usually surgically removed. Certain dietary changes, as well as taking nutritional supplements, may decrease the likelihood of cancer developing elsewhere in the intestines. See also CANCER PREVENTION; RECTAL CANCER.

SUPPLEMENTS

- Calcium: 500–1,000 mg daily (older women: 1,500–2,000 mg).
- Folic acid: 400–800 mcg daily.

HERBS

- Psyllium: as directed on label.

CONSIDER / TRY TO

- Eat more fresh fruits and vegetables.
- Eat oat fiber.
- Eat soy foods, including soy shakes.

AVOID / WATCH OUT FOR

- High-fat foods.
- Low-fiber foods.

Constipation

Constipation—uncomfortable, infrequent bowel movements—can be either an acute or a chronic condition. The causes of acute constipation can include taking prescription drugs, recent inactivity, or a change in dietary habits. Chronic constipation can be caused by any number of conditions, but is most often due to a lack of dietary fiber. Constipation responds well to nutritional supplements and moderate lifestyle changes. See also DIGESTIVE DISORDERS.

CONSTIPATION

SUPPLEMENTS

- Magnesium: 250–500 mg daily.
- Probiotics: one to three capsules *or* one tablespoon of refrigerated liquid probiotics, up to three times daily before meals; *or* acidophilus: one to three (multi-billion count) capsules before meals.
- Vitamin C: 500–1,000 mg daily.

HERBS

- Aloe vera juice: one tablespoon twice daily.
- Cascara sagrada: as directed on label.
- Flaxseed oil (refrigerated): one teaspoon of the oil; *or* 500 mg, one to three times daily (as capsules).
- Psyllium: as directed on label.
- Senna: as directed on label.

CONSIDER / TRY TO

- Detoxification (see TOXICITY on page 280).
- Drink six to eight glasses of pure water daily.
- Eat more fresh vegetables and fruits.
- Eat prunes and bran.
- Exercise regularly.

AVOID / WATCH OUT FOR

- Extended travel.
- Iron supplements.
- Prescription drugs.
- Sugar, cheese, and refined white flour.

Cough

COUGH

Coughing is an attempt by the body to protect the lungs. Coughs can have many causes, ranging from allergies, respiratory infection, and bronchitis to lung cancer, pneumonia, and tuberculosis. Simple coughing, associated with the common cold for example, can be soothed naturally without the need for commonly used over-the-counter cough medicines.

SUPPLEMENTS

- Magnesium: 250–500 mg daily.
- NAC (N-acetylcysteine): 1,500 mg with meals (for bronchitis).
- Vitamin A: 5,000–10,000 IU daily.
- Vitamin C: 500–1,000 mg daily.
- Vitamin E: 400–500 IU daily.

HERBS

- Chickweed: as directed on the label.
- Ginger root tea: drink daily.
- Licorice root: 450 mg, one to three times daily (as capsules).
- Mullein: as directed on label.

CONSIDER / TRY TO

- Clean the ventilation system in your home and office.
- Homeopathic cough remedy.
- Humidifier.

AVOID / WATCH OUT FOR

- Candidiasis.
- Cigarette smoke.
- Dust.
- Excess sugar consumption.

Cystitis

A bladder infection (cystitis) is a lower urinary tract infection caused by bacteria. Bladder infections are more common in women than in men. Symptoms include an urgent, frequent desire to urinate and pain during urination. There may also be lower back pain and pain above the pubic bone. Antibiotics are often prescribed for bladder infections; however, this infection responds very well to natural remedies. See also URINARY TRACT INFECTION.

SUPPLEMENTS

- Complete all-natural multivitamin/mineral complex rich in antioxidants.

HERBS

- Acidophilus: one to three (multi-billion count) capsules before each meal.
- Alfalfa: as directed on label.
- Barberry: as directed on label.
- Cinnamon: as directed on label.
- Cranberry extract: as directed on label (as capsules).
- Garlic: 500 mg daily.
- Uva ursi: as directed on label.

CONSIDER / TRY TO

- Drink six to ten glasses of pure water daily.
- Drink two 8-ounce glasses of unsweetened cranberry juice daily.
- Wear cotton undergarments.

AVOID / WATCH OUT FOR

- Beans.
- Chocolate.
- Feminine hygiene sprays.
- Refined carbohydrates and sugar.
- Talcum powder.

Dandruff

Dandruff, those annoying flakes of skin that fall from the scalp, is actually part of a skin condition known as seborrheic dermatitis. The face and occasionally other areas of the body can also be affected. While topical medications and prescription shampoos are often prescribed for this condition, dandruff can easily be remedied naturally. Quite often, simple dietary changes and nutritional supplementation are all that's required.

SUPPLEMENTS

- Biotin: 300 mcg daily.
- Folic acid: 400–800 mcg daily.
- Kelp: 150 mcg daily.
- Selenium: 100–200 mcg daily.
- Vitamin B_6 (pyridoxine): 25–50 mg daily.
- Vitamin B_{12}: 100–1,000 mcg daily.
- Vitamin E: 400–500 IU daily.
- Zinc: 15 mg of elemental zinc (read label), once or twice daily.

HERBS

- Dandelion: as directed on label.
- Flaxseed oil (refrigerated): one teaspoon of the oil; *or* 500 mg, one to three times daily (as capsules).
- Goldenseal: as directed on label.

CONSIDER / TRY TO

- Eat more fish.
- Eat more raw fruits and vegetables.
- Eat yogurt with live cultures.

AVOID / WATCH OUT FOR

- Dairy products.
- Greasy lotions.
- Irritating shampoo or soaps.
- Nuts, sugar, and fried foods.

Depression

Depression is not merely the blues. It's a serious mood disorder that can have many contributing causes, which aren't fully understood. While it's normal to feel sad occasionally, depression is a lingering, intense sadness that can persist for months or years. Antidepressant drugs are commonly prescribed for depression but carry with them many side effects. Natural remedies can help improve mood and eventually restore a balanced feeling of well-being.

SUPPLEMENTS

- DHEA: 25 mg daily for women over forty; 50 mg daily for men over forty.
- Magnesium: 250–500 mg daily.
- Pregnenolone: 10 mg daily.
- Vitamin B complex: 25–50 mg daily.

HERBS

- Licorice root: 450 mg, one to three times daily (as capsules).
- St. John's wort (dual action): 300 mg, once or twice daily.

CONSIDER / TRY TO

- Detoxification (see TOXICITY on page 280).
- Exercise regularly.
- Get sufficient sleep.
- Participate in a sport.

AVOID / WATCH OUT FOR

- Antidepressant drugs and other prescription drugs.
- "Diet" products and extreme dieting.
- Processed foods.
- Too little dietary fat.

Diabetes

Diabetes mellitus is a condition in which the body either doesn't produce enough insulin to keep blood sugar at normal levels (type 1, or insulin-dependent diabetes), or the cells do not properly respond to the insulin (type 2, or non–insulin-dependent diabetes). While diabetes is a serious condition that has many long-term complications, it is possible to take natural steps under a doctor's supervision to stabilize blood sugar levels and improve the overall condition.

SUPPLEMENTS

- Alpha lipoic acid: 50 mg daily.
- Chromium: 200–600 mg daily.
- Magnesium: 250–500 mg daily.
- MSM: 1,000 mg, one to three times daily.
- Vanadium (Vanadyl): 10 mg daily.
- Vitamin B$_6$ (pyridoxine): 25–50 mg daily.
- Vitamin E: 400–500 IU daily.

HERBS

- Banaba leaf extract: 60 mg at the end of each meal.
- Bilberry extract: as directed on label.
- Garlic: 500 mg daily.
- Ginkgo biloba extract: 60 mg, one to three times daily.

CONSIDER / TRY TO

- Drink six to ten glasses of pure water daily.
- Increase fiber.
- Lose weight if necessary.
- Reduce carbohydrates.

AVOID / WATCH OUT FOR

- Alcohol.
- Low-fiber foods.
- Refined carbohydrates.
- Saturated fats.
- Soft drinks.
- Sugary desserts.

Diarrhea

DIARRHEA

Frequent watery bowel movements accompanied by powerful cramping, commonly known as diarrhea, can be a symptom of many different conditions, including gastroenteritis, irritable bowel syndrome, ulcerative colitis, infection with the salmonella bacteria, and so on. Diarrhea that persists for more than a few days or recurs often should be brought to a doctor's attention; however, occasional bouts with diarrhea can be treated naturally and quite easily at home. See also DIGESTIVE DISORDERS.

SUPPLEMENTS

- Acidophilus: one to three (multi-billion count) capsules before each meal.
- Calcium: 500–1,000 mg daily (older women: 1,500–2,000 mg).
- Digestive enzymes: one to three capsules with each meal.
- Kelp: 150 mcg daily.
- Potassium: 99 mg, one to three times daily.

HERBS

- Chamomile tea: drink three times daily.
- Garlic: 500 mg daily.
- Raspberry leaves tea: drink three times daily.

CONSIDER / TRY TO

- Drink pure water in excess of six to eight glasses daily.
- Eat fresh fruit and vegetables, including carrots.
- Eat more fiber.
- Eat more whole grains.
- Eat yogurt with live cultures.

AVOID / WATCH OUT FOR

- Dairy products.
- Excess magnesium.

Digestive Disorders

The mouth, throat, esophagus, stomach, small and large intestines, rectum, and anus comprise the digestive tract. Some organs outside the digestive tract—the liver, gallbladder, and pancreas—are actually part of the digestive system. Digestive disorders include any malfunction in any part of the digestive system; however, gastritis, a disorder of the stomach, is a common complaint. This condition, of which there are several causes, can quite often be relieved by taking certain supplements and drinking plenty of water. See also CONSTIPATION; DIARRHEA; ULCER, PEPTIC.

SUPPLEMENTS

- Acidophilus: one to three (multi-billion count) capsules before each meal.
- Digestive enzymes: one to three capsules with each meal.
- MSM: 1,000 mg, one to three times daily.
- Potassium: 99 mg, one to three times daily.

HERBS

- No herbs apply.

CONSIDER / TRY TO

- Drink six to eight glasses of pure water daily.

Diverticulosis/Diverticulitis

Abnormal sacs that develop in the large intestine are known as diverticula. Quite common in the elderly, diverticulosis is the condition of having many diverticula. Although the exact cause is unknown, a long-term diet lacking in sufficient fiber and water may play a role. When waste becomes trapped in the diverticula, it can lead to inflammation and infection. This more serious condition is known as diverticulitis. However, before the diverticula become inflamed, it is possible to improve the condition and avoid infection by following some basic dietary guidelines and taking nutritional supplements.

SUPPLEMENTS

• Apple pectin: 500 mg daily.
• Glutamine: 50–150 mg daily.
• MSM: 1,000 mg, three times daily.
• Prebiotic fiber supplement: as directed on label.

HERBS

• Aloe vera extract: one tablespoon, twice daily.
• Cat's claw: 500 mg, one to three times daily
  (as capsules).
• Grape seed extract: 200 mg daily.
• Green tea extract: 200 mg daily.

CONSIDER / TRY TO

• Drink peppermint tea.
• Dump an entire box of Epsom salts in a hot bath.
  Your bowels will be moving again within a few
  hours.
• Eat generous amounts of garlic and onions.
• Eat more fiber, including fresh fruits and vegetables.
• Eat plain, unsweetened yogurt daily.
• Exercise.

AVOID / WATCH OUT FOR

• Caffeine.
• Dairy products.
• Drugs that can cause constipation, such as diuretics,
  painkillers, tranquilizers, antidepressants,
  antihistamines, narcotics, and decongestants.
• Large meals. Eat smaller meals more frequently.

Dry Eye Syndrome

Quite common among Americans, dry eye syndrome is usually caused by inadequate tear production. While there are many causes of dry eye syndrome, the aging process is the most common culprit. Other contributing causes include hot, dry, or windy climates; high altitudes; cigarette smoke; air conditioning; reading; and working on a computer. Resting or blinking the eyes periodically may help comfort them. In addition to other natural remedies, drinking eight to ten 8-ounce glasses of water a day helps hydrate the body and flush impurities.

DRY EYE SYNDROME

SUPPLEMENTS

- Evening primrose oil: 500 mg, three times daily.
- MSM: 1,000 mg, three times daily.

HERBS

- Bilberry extract: 60 mg, twice daily.
- Ginkgo biloba: 60 mg, twice daily.
- Grape seed extract: 200 mg daily.
- Green tea extract: 200 mg daily.
- Omega-3 fatty acids: 1,000 mg daily (as fish oil capsules).

CONSIDER / TRY TO

- Drink eight to ten glasses of pure water daily.
- Eat foods rich in omega-3 fatty acids, such as salmon, tuna, herring, and cod, twice weekly.
- Exercise regularly.
- Reduce stress.
- Replace contact lenses with eye glasses.
- Wear UV-blocking sunglasses.

AVOID / WATCH OUT FOR

- Alcohol.
- Caffeine.
- Exposing your eyes to high temperatures.
- Processed foods, especially sugar, white flour, and other refined carbohydrates.
- Smoking.

Dry Skin

Dry skin affects people of all ages, but it is especially common in those who are past middle age. Cold weather and frequent bathing are common causes. Also, harsh soaps, detergents, and perfumes tend to dry out the skin and/or exacerbate the problem. One of the most successful remedies is keeping the skin moist. Ointments and creams can help since they hold water in the skin. Proper nutrition and adequate water intake are also very important in maintaining moist, firm skin.

SUPPLEMENTS

- Complete all-natural multivitamin/mineral complex rich in antioxidants.
- Evening primrose oil: 500 mg, two to three times daily.
- MSM: 1,000 mg, three times daily.

HERBS

- Burdock root: 500 mg, one to two times daily (as capsules).
- Flaxseed oil: 1,000 mg daily.
- Grape seed extract: 200 mg daily.
- Green tea extract: 200 mg daily.
- Omega-3 fatty acids: 1,000 mg daily (as fish oil capsules).
- Silica: 30 mg daily.

CONSIDER / TRY TO

- Avoid commercial cosmetics, soaps, and skin and facial creams.
- Brush your skin with a loofah sponge daily.
- Drink eight to ten glasses of pure water daily.
- Eat foods rich in omega-3 fatty acids, such as salmon, tuna, herring, and cod, twice weekly.
- Eat plain, unsweetened yogurt daily.
- Test for allergies.
- Test for low thyroid.

AVOID / WATCH OUT FOR

- Alcohol.
- Caffeine.
- Fried foods.
- Hot baths and showers.
- Processed foods and foods high in trans fatty acids.

Ear Infection

Pain in the ear can be caused by any number of factors, including bacteria, injury, fluid buildup, and accumulated pus. The outer ear, middle ear, or inner ear may be affected. Ear infections that are caused by bacteria, such as "swimmer's ear," are commonly treated with antibiotics. Nutritional and herbal supplements, however, are very effective at clearing up ear infections without any of the side effects associated with antibiotics.

SUPPLEMENTS

- Acidophilus: one to three (multi-billion count) capsules before each meal.
- Complete all-natural multivitamin/mineral complex rich in antioxidants.

HERBS

- Echinacea: as directed on label.
- Garlic: 500 mg daily.

CONSIDER / TRY TO

- Eat soy products.
- Liquid garlic, warmed and dropped into ear canal; plug with cotton for 10 to 15 minutes.

AVOID / WATCH OUT FOR

- Dairy products.
- Excessive use of antibiotics.

Eczema, Atopic

ECZEMA, ATOPIC

Any inflammation of the skin is known as
dermatitis. There are many types and causes
of dermatitis. *Atopic* eczema, a type of atopic
dermatitis, is a chronic, hereditary condition in
which patches of the skin become red, dry,
and excessively itchy. Scratching the affected
areas exacerbates the problem and can lead
to infection. When a flare-up is particularly bad,
corticosteroids are often prescribed, but with
little success at preventing future flare-ups.
Fortunately, natural remedies can successfully
heal the affected skin and reduce the overall
severity of the condition.

SUPPLEMENTS

- Complete all-natural multivitamin/mineral complex rich in antioxidants.
- Evening primrose oil: 500 mg, two to three times daily.
- Flaxseed oil: 1,000 mg daily.
- Glutamine: 50–150 mg daily.
- MSM: 1,000 mg, three times daily.
- Prebiotic fiber blend: as directed on label.
- Zinc: 15 mg of elemental zinc, once or twice daily.

HERBS

- Burdock: as directed on label.
- Grape seed extract: 200 mg daily.
- Green tea extract: 200 mg daily.
- Silica: 30 mg daily.

CONSIDER / TRY TO

- Drink eight to ten glasses of pure water daily.
- Eat foods rich in omega-3 fatty acids twice weekly.
- Eat plain, unsweetened yogurt daily.
- Exercise regularly.
- For babies, try breastfeeding instead of bottle feeding.
- Reduce stress.
- Take herbal baths using chamomile, lavender, and oatmeal.
- Test for low thyroid.

AVOID / WATCH OUT FOR

- Alcohol.
- Caffeine.
- Exposure to extreme temperatures—hot or cold.
- Extremely hot baths or showers and excessive bathing.
- Foods rich in trans fatty acids.
- Fried or processed foods.

Emotional/Physical Lows

It's perfectly normal to sometimes feel sad, tired, agitated, anxious, and so on. And it isn't always obvious why you're feeling that way. While there are a number of prescription drugs to counteract your negative feelings—whether they are physical or emotional—a much better and safer way to improve your condition is to inhale the essences of essential oils. Whatever the desired outcome, within moments of inhalation, you should begin feeling better. See AROMATHERAPY on page 306.

EMOTIONAL/PHYSICAL LOWS

AROMATHERAPY FOR
EMOTIONAL/PHYSICAL LOWS

If you're feeling...	Try inhaling essence of...	For the effect of...
Agitated	Bergamot	Restfulness
Anxious	Catnip	Calmness
Forgetful	Lily of the valley	Improved memory
Inner turmoil	Lily	Inner peace
Sad	Apple	Cheerfulness
Unable to sleep	Hops	Sleepiness
Unclean	Hyssop	Purification
Unenergetic	Camphor, ginger, or saffron	Increased energy
Uninterested in sex	Cardamom	Increased sexual desire
Uninterested in sex and loving feelings	Vanilla	Sex and love
Unloved or unloving	Jasmine	Love
Wounded	Eucalyptus or myrrh	Healing

Emphysema

Emphysema is the irreversible damage and
enlargement of the air sacs of the lungs,
causing a decreased rate of airflow. Cigarette
smoking is the most common cause of
emphysema. Symptoms include shortness
of breath or wheezing. Keeping the immune
system strong by not smoking, eating a healthy
diet, and taking nutritional supplements, as
well as avoiding exposure to airborne irritants,
including secondhand smoke and air pollution,
may help delay and ease the symptoms.

SUPPLEMENTS

- Complete all-natural multivitamin/mineral complex rich in antioxidants.
- Evening primrose oil: 500 mg, two to three times daily.
- Glutamine: 50–150 mg daily.
- MSM: 1,000 mg, three times daily.
- N-Acetyl-cysteine: 500 mg, twice daily.
- Zinc: 15 mg of elemental zinc daily.

HERBS

- Astragalus: 200 mg, three times daily.
- Ginkgo biloba: 60 mg, twice daily.
- Grape seed extract: 200 mg daily.
- Green tea extract: 200 mg daily.

CONSIDER / TRY TO

- An air-filtration system throughout your living quarters and, if possible, a portable one at your home.

AVOID / WATCH OUT FOR

- Air pollution.
- Smoke, including secondhand smoke.

Fatigue

FATIGUE

Simple fatigue, as opposed to chronic fatigue, is usually a result of lifestyle factors that stress the body, such as a lack of sufficient sleep, lack of proper nutrition, strenuous physical activity, and smoking. If it is not accompanied by other symptoms that may indicate a more serious problem, fatigue responds quite well to natural remedies, including getting a sufficient amount of sleep nightly. If persistent fatigue is your problem, see also CHRONIC FATIGUE SYNDROME (CFS).

SUPPLEMENTS

- Coenzyme Q_{10}: 60 mg, one to three times daily.
- DHEA: 25 mg daily for women over age 40; 50 mg daily for men over age 40.
- Pregnenolone: 10 mg daily.
- Selenium: 100–200 mcg daily.

HERBS

- Astragalus: as directed on label.
- Buplerum: as directed on label.
- Ginseng: as directed on label.
- Grape seed/green tea complex: 100 mg of each twice daily.

CONSIDER / TRY TO

- Acupuncture.
- Detoxification (see TOXICITY on page 280).
- Exercise regularly.

AVOID / WATCH OUT FOR

- Adrenal exhaustion.
- Candida Infection.
- Environmental toxins.
- Estrogen dominance.
- Food allergens.
- Synthetic hormones (birth control pills and HRT).

Fibromyalgia

Fibromyalgia is a syndrome characterized by chronic pain and stiffness in the muscles, tendons, and ligaments, occurring throughout the body, or sometimes in only one specific area or areas. Pressure to certain spots on the body may cause pain. While the cause of fibromyalgia remains unknown, triggers may include stress, lack of sleep, injury, or infection. It's not necessary to turn to prescription medication for relief, as this condition can be treated naturally.

SUPPLEMENTS

- Arginine, timed-release: 1,500 mg twice daily.
- Coenzyme Q_{10}: 60 mg, one to three times daily.
- Evening primrose oil: 500–1,000 mg daily (as capsules).
- MSM (with vitamin C complex): one tablet, three times daily.
- Vitamin E: 400–500 IU daily.

HERBS

- Cayenne: as directed on label.
- Ginger extract (EV EXT 77): one capsule, three times daily with food.
- Grape seed/green tea complex: 100 mg of each twice daily.

CONSIDER / TRY TO

- Acupressure.
- Biofeedback.
- Massage.
- Yoga.

AVOID / WATCH OUT FOR

- Alcohol.
- Caffeine.
- Excess sugar and salt.
- Stress.
- Tobacco.

Fungal Skin Infections

Fungi—of which there are various types in the plant kingdom—are prevalent in our environment. Certain types of fungi can infect the topmost layer (or dead layer) of the skin, causing conditions such as ringworm. Symptoms can range from redness and mild scaling and itching to extremely irritated, blistered skin. Although fungi are difficult to eradicate, natural remedies work well when used for three to six months. See also ATHLETE'S FOOT; CANDIDIASIS.

FUNGAL SKIN INFECTIONS

SUPPLEMENTS

- Acidophilus: one to three (multi-billion count) capsules before each meal.
- Vitamin B complex: 25–50 mg daily.
- Vitamin C: 500–1,000 mg daily.
- Vitamin E: 400–500 IU daily.
- Zinc: 15 mg of elemental zinc (read label), once or twice daily.

HERBS

- Garlic: 500 mg daily.
- Grapefruit seed extract: as directed on label.
- Tea tree oil: apply topically as directed on label.

CONSIDER / TRY TO

- Eat more raw fruits and vegetables.
- Keep infected areas dry.

AVOID / WATCH OUT FOR

- Reduce consumption of meat, grains, and dairy.

Gallstones

Gallstones are crystallized masses of mostly cholesterol that develop in the gallbladder. However, they can also travel to, or occur in, the bile ducts. As long as the stones remain in the gallbladder, this condition can remain silent for many years, or pain of various degrees may come and go. If a gallstone completely obstructs a duct, serious complications can occur. If you're prone to gallstones, there are many natural ways you can reduce the risk of further development.

SUPPLEMENTS

- Lecithin granules: one tablespoon, one to three times daily.
- Taurine: 500–1,500 mg daily.

HERBS

- Dandelion: as directed on label.
- Milk thistle (silymarin): 140 mg, one to three times daily (as capsules).
- Peppermint: as directed on label.
- Turmeric: as directed on label.

CONSIDER / TRY TO

- Eat oat bran.
- Vegetarian diet.

AVOID / WATCH OUT FOR

- Low-fiber foods.
- Refined carbohydrates.
- Saturated fats.

Gas, Intestinal

While it's normal for a person to pass gas relatively often throughout the day, excessive intestinal gas—that is, frequent flatulence—can be quite uncomfortable and, sometimes, embarrassing. The amount of intestinal gas a person has is generally related to the diet. For example, a person who cannot properly digest lactose (milk sugars) will find that he or she is beset with excessive gas after drinking a glass of milk. Avoiding offending foods is obviously key here, but there are other natural steps that can be taken to reduce the production of gas and/or provide relief in the case of bloating.

SUPPLEMENTS

- Charcoal tablets: one with each meal. Do NOT take for more than three consecutive days.
- Digestive enzymes (plant based): one to three times with each meal (as capsules).
- MSM (with vitamin C complex): 1,000 mg, three times daily.
- Prebiotic fiber blend: as directed on label.

HERBS

- Garlic extract: 500 mg, one to two times daily (as odorless capsules).
- Ginger extract (EV EXT 77): 170 mg, one to three times daily with meals.

CONSIDER / TRY TO

- Anise seeds sprinkled on salad.
- Eat a slice of pineapple before meals.
- Eat slowly and chew your food completely.
- Use Beano.

AVOID / WATCH OUT FOR

- Alcohol.
- Caffeine.
- Chewing gum.
- Gas-producing foods, such as beans or dairy products (except for plain, unsweetened yogurt).
- Processed foods.
- Soft drinks or other carbonated beverages.
- Stress.
- Sugar substitutes, such as sorbitol and manitol.

Gingivitis

Inflammation of the gums is known as gingivitis. The main cause of this condition is plaque buildup along the gum line. Symptoms include red, swollen gums that bleed easily. While brushing and flossing regularly can prevent gum disease, other natural steps—such as including nutritional supplements in your daily regimen—can be taken to improve the condition of your gums.

SUPPLEMENTS

- Beta-carotene: 10,000–20,000 IU daily.
- Coenzyme Q_{10}: 60 mg, one to three times daily.
- Copper: 2–3 mg daily.
- Folic acid: 400–800 mcg daily.
- Selenium: 100–200 mcg daily.
- Vitamin C: 500–1,000 mg daily.
- Vitamin E: 400–500 IU daily.
- Zinc: 15 mg of elemental zinc (read label), once or twice daily.

HERBS

- Hawthorne extract: as directed on label.
- Quercetin: 400 mg before eating, one to three times daily.
- Tea tree oil toothpaste: brush regularly.

CONSIDER / TRY TO

- Brush and floss regularly.
- Eat foods high in fiber.
- Eat raw, crunchy vegetables.
- Rinse mouth with mixture of hydrogen peroxide and water.
- Use toothpicks.
- Water irrigation/stimulation.

AVOID / WATCH OUT FOR

- All simple sugars.
- Excess alcohol.
- Refined carbohydrates.
- Smoking.

Glaucoma

Glaucoma is a group of eye diseases characterized by increased pressure in the eyeball, leading to damage of the optic nerve. This damage results in gradual vision loss and, if not treated, can lead to total blindness. Open-angle glaucoma is the most common form, and affects mostly older adults. Secondary glaucoma is a complication of other disorders, such as diabetes. Routine eye examinations by an eye-care professional generally include a test for glaucoma. When caught early, measures can be taken, including the remedies listed here, to reduce the pressure and thereby avoid vision loss.

SUPPLEMENTS

- Alpha lipoic acid: 50 mg daily.
- L-Arginine: 1,500 mg, twice daily (as timed-release capsule).
- MSM (with vitamin C complex): 1,000 mg, three times daily.
- Zinc: 15 mg of elemental zinc daily.

HERBS

- Bilberry extract: 60 mg, twice daily.
- Ginkgo biloba: 60 mg, twice daily.
- Grape seed extract: 200 mg daily.
- Green tea extract: 200 mg daily.

CONSIDER / TRY TO

- Drink eight to ten glasses of pure water daily.
- Eat foods rich in omega-3 fatty acids, twice weekly.
- Eat plenty of fresh fruits and vegetables.
- Limit your intake of dairy products.
- Maintain a healthy body weight.
- Wear quality sunglasses when exposed to sun for prolonged periods.

AVOID / WATCH OUT FOR

- Alcohol.
- Caffeine.
- Cortisone drugs.
- Excessive exposure to sun.
- Eye strain.
- Smoking and breathing secondhand smoke.
- Stress.

Gout

Gout is a painful condition in which excess uric acid crystallizes in a joint or joints and causes inflammation (arthritis). Joints commonly affected include those in the feet, knees, wrists, and elbows. Dietary factors, such as high-protein consumption, may play a role in the development of this condition. Natural remedies are aimed at ridding the body of excess uric acid and reducing inflammation.

SUPPLEMENTS

- MSM: 1,000 mg, one to three times daily.
- Multiple antioxidant formula: as directed on label.
- Vitamin B complex: 25–50 mg daily.
- Vitamin B_6 (pyridoxine): 25–50 mg daily.

HERBS

- Celery juice: drink daily.
- Cherry juice: drink daily.
- Ginger extract (EV EXT 77): 170 mg, one to two times daily (as capsules).
- Grape seed extract (PCOs): 100 mg, one to three times daily.

CONSIDER / TRY TO

- Drink six to eight glasses of pure water daily.
- Reduce protein intake.

AVOID / WATCH OUT FOR

- Excess protein.
- High-purine food, such as organ meats, scallops, mussels, sardines, and herring.

Hair Loss

Hair loss—in this case, the loss of hair on the head—has a number of causes, including male-pattern baldness, improper hair care, alopecia areata (patchy or complete hair loss), childbirth, chemotherapy, medication, inadequate nutrition, and so on. In many cases, hair loss is temporary and will correct itself when the cause is removed. While some hair loss is irreversible, the loss of hair can be slowed and the condition can be improved by making sure to eat a nutrient-rich diet accompanied by certain hair-healthy supplements.

SUPPLEMENTS

- Beta sitosterol: 60 mg, twice daily.
- Biotin: 1,000 mcg daily.
- Choline and inositol: 1,000 mg daily.
- Cysteine: 1,000 mg daily.

HERBS

- Fo-ti: as directed on label.
- Parsley oil: apply topically to affected area.
- Saw palmetto: 150 mg, twice daily for men and women.

CONSIDER / TRY TO

- Drink eight to ten glasses of pure water daily.
- Eat a high-protein diet.
- Massage the scalp three times daily.
- Rinse your hair with apple cider or sage tea occasionally.

AVOID / WATCH OUT FOR

- Blow dryers (towel dry instead).
- Commercial shampoos or rinses with artificial colors, preservatives, and dyes.
- Hair spray.

Hair, Skin, and Nail Problems

Hair, skin, and nail problems often occur simultaneously. For example, hair and nails may become dry and brittle, while at the same time the skin becomes dry and flaky. Or hair and skin may become oily, while the nails become soft. Whatever the symptoms, inadequate nutrition is often the culprit in these conditions. It's easy to remedy these problems naturally so that hair regains its glossiness, skin its suppleness, and nails their hardness.

HAIR, SKIN, AND NAIL PROBLEMS

SUPPLEMENTS

- Biotin: 300 mcg daily.
- Calcium: 500–1,000 mg daily (older women: 1,500–2,000 mg).
- Kelp: 150 mcg daily.
- L-Cysteine: 100–250 mg, one to two times daily.
- Magnesium: 250–500 mg daily.
- Selenium: 100–200 mcg daily.
- Vitamin C: 500–1,000 mg daily.
- Vitamin E: 400–500 IU daily.
- Zinc: 15 mg of elemental zinc (read label), once or twice daily.

HERBS

- Aloe vera gel: apply topically as directed on label.
- Dandelion: as directed on label.
- Evening primrose oil: 500 mg, one to three times daily.
- Horsetail: as directed on the label.
- Oregon grape root: as directed on label.
- Yellow dock: as directed on label.

CONSIDER / TRY TO

- Apply alpha-hydroxy acid to skin as directed on product label.
- Drink six to eight glasses of pure water daily.
- Eat foods high in protein.
- Rinse hair with apple cider or sage tea.
- Wear gloves to protect hands and nails.

AVOID / WATCH OUT FOR

- Excess sun exposure leading to sunburn and/or tanning.
- Excess vitamin A.

Hay Fever

People who suffer from hay fever are allergic to plant pollen. Since trees, grasses, and other plants produce pollen seasonally, hay fever is often referred to as seasonal allergies. Symptoms include sneezing, itchy and watery eyes, and a runny or stuffed nose. When allergy season comes around, many people turn to the widely available prescription and over-the-counter antihistamines, or allergy medicines. What they don't realize is that hay fever can be controlled quite well with natural, time-tested remedies. See also ALLERGIES TO DUST, MOLD, AND DANDER; SINUSITIS.

Hay Fever

SUPPLEMENTS

- Digestive enzymes: one to three capsules with each meal.
- Magnesium: 250–500 mg daily.
- Vitamin B complex: 25–50 mg daily.
- Vitamin C: 500–1,000 mg daily.
- Zinc: 15 mg of elemental zinc (read label), once or twice daily.

HERBS

- Borage oil: 500–1,000 mg daily (as capsules) *or* evening primrose oil: 500–1,000 mg daily (as capsules).
- Echinacea: as directed on label.
- Ginkgo biloba extract: 60 mg, one to three times daily.
- Grape seed extract (PCOs): 100 mg, one to three times daily.
- Licorice root: 450 mg, one to three times daily (as capsules).
- Quercetin: 400 mg before eating, one to three times daily.

CONSIDER / TRY TO

- Colon-cleansing program.
- Detoxification (see TOXICITY on page 280).
- Drink pure water in excess of six to eight glasses daily.
- Immune-system boosters (see IMMUNE SYSTEM, WEAKENED on page 164).

AVOID / WATCH OUT FOR

- Pollen.

Headaches

Some people get headaches frequently, others get them rarely, but virtually everyone has experienced the characteristic throbbing sensation. The causes of headaches vary, and constant recurrence may indicate an underlying condition. However, headaches often have relatively minor causes, such as tension. Relief of a headache can come quite quickly—without the use of aspirin, ibuprofen, acetaminophen, and so on. Common herbs and other natural steps not only bring relief of the actual headache but also may reduce their frequency. See also MIGRAINES.

SUPPLEMENTS

- Calcium: 500–1,000 mg daily (older women: 1,500–2,000 mg).
- DLPA (dl-phenylalanine): 375–750 mg, every four hours for discomfort (as capsules).
- Magnesium: 250–500 mg daily.
- Niacin (vitamin B_3): 50–1,000 mg daily, in divided doses.
- Pantothenic acid (vitamin B_5): 30–100 mg daily.
- Vitamin C: 500–1,000 mg daily.
- Vitamin E: 400–500 IU daily.

HERBS

- Chamomile tea: drink one cup daily.
- Feverfew: as directed on label.
- Ginkgo biloba extract: 60 mg, one to three times daily.
- Thyme tea: drink one cup daily.
- White willow bark: 500–1,000 mg, two to three times daily (as capsules).

CONSIDER / TRY TO

- Acupuncture or acupressure.
- Cold compress made with basil tea and witch hazel, applied to forehead.
- Drink six to eight glasses of pure water daily.
- Exercise moderately.
- Massage.

AVOID / WATCH OUT FOR

- Food additives, such as MSG.
- Food allergies.
- Pollen, dust, and environmental toxins.
- Red meat, nuts, chocolate, coffee, and wine.

Hearing Loss

Hearing loss—a deterioration in hearing (as opposed to deafness, which is defined as profound hearing loss)—can have a number of different causes, such as exposure to very loud noise, taking certain drugs, Ménière's disease, stroke, and some hereditary diseases. A buildup of earwax or fluid can also be the culprit. While hearing loss is often irreversible, further deterioration can be avoided by taking protective nutritional supplements and by following some commonsense advice.

SUPPLEMENTS

- Magnesium: 250–500 mg daily.
- Niacin (vitamin B$_3$): 50–1,000 mg daily, in divided doses.
- Vitamin B$_{12}$: 100–1,000 mcg daily.

HERBS

- Ginkgo biloba extract: 60 mg, one to three times daily.

CONSIDER / TRY TO

- Wear protective headphones/earplugs.

AVOID / WATCH OUT FOR

- Loud noises and music.

Heartburn

Virtually everyone has experienced the pain of heartburn at least once in his or her life, often as a result of eating too much or too fast. Defined as a burning pain behind the breastbone, heartburn is caused by acid reflux, the backflow of stomach contents upward into the esophagus. The pain, which rises in the chest, may extend into the neck, throat, or even face. If you're a frequent sufferer of heartburn, there are a number of natural remedies that you can use to help prevent further occurrences.

SUPPLEMENTS

- Acidophilus: one to three (multi-billion count) capsules before each meal.
- Betaine hydrochloride (HCL): 150 mg with each meal (as capsules).
- Digestive enzymes: one to three capsules with each meal.
- Vitamin B_{12}: 100–1,000 mcg daily.

HERBS

- Aloe vera juice: one tablespoon twice daily.
- Papaya: one to three tablets after a meal or eat the fruit after a large meal.
- Slippery elm: as directed on label.

CONSIDER / TRY TO

- After eating, stay upright; take a walk.
- Drink a glass of room-temperature water before meals.
- Eat smaller meals slowly.
- Lose excess weight.

AVOID / WATCH OUT FOR

- Antacids.
- Foods and beverages known to trigger heartburn.
- Prescription H2 Blockers, such as Zantac.
- Smoking.

Hemorrhoids

Hemorrhoids are inflamed veins in the wall of the rectum or anus. They can sometimes be painful and occasionally may bleed. Straining during bowel movements is the main cause of this condition. Natural remedies are aimed at relieving pain and reducing inflammation as well as improving the ease of bowel movements.

SUPPLEMENTS

- Acidophilus: one to three (multi-billion count) capsules before each meal.
- Fiber supplement: four tablets, twice daily.
- Rutin: 50 mg, one to three times daily.
- Vitamin C: 500–1,000 mg daily with 500 mg of bioflavonoids daily.
- Vitamin E oil or cream: apply to hemorrhoid.

HERBS

- No herbs apply.

CONSIDER / TRY TO

- Drink six to ten glasses of pure water daily.
- Eat unprocessed bran.
- Exercise regularly.

AVOID / WATCH OUT FOR

- Coffee, chocolate, cola, and cocoa.

Hepatitis

Hepatitis is any inflammation of the liver. It
is caused by a number of different hepatitis
viruses—hepatitis A, B, C, D, and E—each with
its own method of transmission. When liver
inflammation persists for more than six months,
it is said to be a chronic condition. Chronic
hepatitis, which often has no outward symptoms,
can eventually lead to cirrhosis (see page 86).
Natural therapies are aimed at supporting the
liver and helping to reduce liver inflammation
in its early stages.

SUPPLEMENTS

- Complete all-natural multivitamin/mineral complex rich in antioxidants.
- Glutamine: 50–150 mg daily.
- Prebiotic fiber blend: as directed on label.

HERBS

- Dandelion extract: as directed on label.
- Garlic extract: 500 mg, twice daily.
- Grape seed extract: 200 mg daily.
- Green tea extract: 200 mg daily.
- Milk thistle seed extract: 200 mg, three times daily.

CONSIDER / TRY TO

- Drink eight to ten glasses of pure water daily.
- Drink several cups of green tea daily.
- Exercise regularly.
- Increase consumption of fresh fruits and vegetables.
- Reduce stress.

AVOID / WATCH OUT FOR

- Alcohol.
- Caffeine.
- Prescription and over-the-counter drugs unless absolutely necessary.
- Smoking and breathing secondhand smoke.
- Tattoos and body piercing.

Herpes, Genital

Genital herpes is a sexually transmitted disease. Although type II herpes is the common cause of genital herpes, the herpes virus that causes cold sores (type I) can also infect the genitals, and vice versa. The initial infection is quite often the most painful and may last for several weeks before complete healing occurs. Thereafter, the virus remains dormant in the body until it is reactivated and causes an outbreak. Natural remedies are aimed at reducing the frequency of outbreaks and reducing the duration of an outbreak if one occurs.

SUPPLEMENTS

- Complete all-natural multivitamin/mineral complex rich in antioxidants.
- L-Lysine: 500 mg, three times daily between meals.
- MSM: 1,000 mg, three times daily.
- Selenium: 200 mcg daily.

HERBS

- Astragalus: 400 mg, twice daily.
- Grape seed: 200 mg daily.
- Green tea: 200 mg daily.
- Olive leaf extract: 500 mg, twice daily.

CONSIDER / TRY TO

- Apply lemon balm or MSM therapeutic lotion to areas affected.
- Eat plain, unsweetened yogurt daily.
- Eat generous amounts of fresh garlic, onions, shiitake and reishi mushrooms daily.
- Increase consumption of fresh fruits and vegetables.

AVOID / WATCH OUT FOR

- Alcohol.
- Caffeine and other drugs.
- Excessive exposure to the sun.
- Smoking or breathing secondhand smoke.

Herpes, Oral

There are two types of the herpes simplex virus—type I and type II. Type I is the cause of cold sores that form on or around the lips, while type II is usually the cause of genital herpes. The characteristic blisters are contagious, and care should be taken to avoid skin-to-skin contact. Between outbreaks, the virus lies dormant in the body. Flare-ups often occur during times of stress. Natural remedies can speed the healing of blisters and reduce the frequency of outbreaks.

SUPPLEMENTS

- Lysine: 500 mg before eating, once daily; therapeutically 3–4 grams (during a breakout).
- Vitamin A: 5,000–10,000 IU daily.
- Vitamin C: 500–1,000 mg daily with 500 mg of bioflavonoids daily.
- Zinc: 15 mg of elemental zinc (read label), once or twice daily.

HERBS

- Arnica homeopathic tablets: dissolve under tongue as directed on label.
- Calendula ointment or gel: apply topically as directed on label.
- Elderberry: as directed on label.
- Licorice root: 450 mg, one to three times daily (as capsules).

CONSIDER / TRY TO

- Topical witch hazel.

AVOID / WATCH OUT FOR

- Chocolate.
- Coffee.
- Nuts.
- Stress.
- Toothpaste with sodium lauryl sulfate (detergent) or sodium laureth sulfate.

Hiccups

Hiccups are repeated spasms of the diaphragm (the muscle that divides the chest and stomach). While frequent or persistent hiccups may indicate an underlying disorder, these spasms are usually harmless. However, as almost anyone will admit, they can be rather bothersome (and perhaps even embarrassing) when they occur. Before you resort to holding your breath yet again, consider natural remedies to ease—and avoid—the problem.

SUPPLEMENTS

- Calcium: 500 mg, twice daily.
- Magnesium: 250 mg daily (as capsules).
- Vitamin B complex: 50 mg, twice daily.

HERBS

Mint leaves: one teaspoon, chew and swallow.

CONSIDER / TRY TO

- Breathe into a paper bag for several minutes.
- Chew and swallow a few slices of fresh ginger.
- Chew and swallow mustard seeds.
- Mix a tablespoon of organic honey in warm water or herbal tea and sip slowly.
- Slowly eat a teaspoon of organic peanut butter.
- Swallow some crushed ice.

AVOID / WATCH OUT FOR

- Eating too quickly.
- Hot, spicy foods or beverages.
- Stress.

Hypoglycemia

Hypoglycemia is a condition in which blood-sugar levels are abnormally low. It is most often found in people with diabetes, as it is a side effect of the diabetic drug insulin. Prolonged fasting or excessive alcohol consumption can, on occasion, also lead to hypoglycemia. Common symptoms of hypoglycemia include sweating, nervousness, faintness, quivering, and, in more serious cases, fatigue, blurry vision, and headaches. Fortunately, many of these symptoms can often be relieved naturally.

SUPPLEMENTS

- Alpha lipoic acid: 50 mg daily.
- Chromium: 200–600 mg daily.
- Essential fatty acids: 250 mg, one to three times daily (as capsules).
- Inositol hexanicotinate (no-flush niacin): 250–500 mg daily.
- MSM: 1,000 mg, one to three times daily.
- Vanadium (Vanadyl): 10 mg daily.
- Vitamin C: 500–1,000 mg daily.
- Vitamin E: 400–500 IU daily.

HERBS

- Banaba leaf extract: 60 mg at the end of each meal.
- Ginkgo biloba extract: 60 mg, one to three times daily.
- Ginseng: as directed on label.
- Grape seed extract (PCOs): 100 mg, one to three times daily.

CONSIDER / TRY TO

- Eat more vegetables.
- Exercise regularly.
- Lose weight if necessary.

AVOID / WATCH OUT FOR

- All sugars and refined carbohydrates.
- Excess carbohydrates.
- Processed foods.

Immune System, Weakened

Your immune system is your body's first line of defense against invaders. When your immune system is not functioning at its peak, you are more prone to infection. Many factors, including stress, contribute to a weakened immune system. Also, when your body is busy fighting off one infection, your immune system may not be strong enough to fight another infection developing elsewhere. So, it's always a good idea to help your immune system along by supplementing a healthy diet with immune boosters, such as vitamins and other natural substances.

IMMUNE SYSTEM, WEAKENED

SUPPLEMENTS

- Beta-carotene: 10,000–20,000 IU daily.
- DHEA: 25 mg daily for women over forty; 50 mg daily for men over forty.
- Glutathione: 50 mg, one to three times daily.
- Melatonin: 1–3 mg, just before bedtime.
- Selenium: 100–200 mcg daily.
- Vitamin B_6 (pyridoxine): 25–50 mg daily.
- Vitamin C: 500–1,000 mg daily.
- Zinc: 15 mg of elemental zinc (read label), once or twice daily.

HERBS

- Astragalus: as directed on label.
- Barberry: as directed on label.
- Echinacea: as directed on label.
- Garlic: 500 mg daily.
- Goldenseal: as directed on label.
- Grape seed/green tea complex: 100 mg of each, twice daily.
- Oregon grape root: as directed on label.
- Osha: as directed on label.

CONSIDER / TRY TO

- Biofeedback.
- Eat vegetables.
- Eat whole foods.
- Eat yogurt with live cultures.
- Exercise regularly.
- Fresh fruit diet.

AVOID / WATCH OUT FOR

- Sugar.
- Stress.

Impotence

Impotence is a condition in which a man cannot get or maintain an erection to carry out intercourse at least half the time sex is attempted. This condition is quite often attributable to underlying physical problems, and can even be a side effect of certain medications. Making some simple lifestyle changes as well as supplementing the diet with nutrients and herbs can go a long way toward remedying this problem.

SUPPLEMENTS

- Arginine: 1,500 mg, twice daily (as timed-release tablets).
- DHEA: 50 mg daily for men over forty.
- Magnesium: 250–500 mg daily.
- Selenium: 100–200 mcg daily.
- Vitamin A: 5,000–10,000 IU daily.
- Vitamin B complex: 25–50 mg daily.
- Vitamin C: 500–1,000 mg daily.
- Vitamin E: 400–500 IU daily.
- Zinc: 15 mg of elemental zinc (read label), once or twice daily.

HERBS

- Ashwagandha: as directed on label.
- Astragalus: as directed on label.
- Avena sativa: as directed on label.
- Ginkgo biloba extract: 60 mg, one to three times daily.
- Ginseng: as directed on label.
- Gotu kola: as directed on label.
- Yohimbe: as directed on label.

CONSIDER / TRY TO

- Cut down on alcohol consumption.
- Cut down on sugar and fat.
- Drink pure water in excess of eight glasses.
- Reduce stress.

AVOID / WATCH OUT FOR

- Hot tubs and saunas.
- Prescription drugs.
- Smoking.
- Too much exercise.

Indigestion

Almost all of us are familiar with the unpleasant
sensation of indigestion, often after we've eaten
a big meal. Indigestion, or dyspepsia, is defined
as a pain or discomfort in the upper abdomen
or chest that's often described as having gas, a
feeling of fullness, or a burning pain. It is usually
a result of something benign, like anxiety, acid
reflux, or lactose intolerance, although it can
sometimes indicate a more serious stomach
problem. The symptoms of indigestion can
usually be treated very effectively using a
regimen of natural remedies.

SUPPLEMENTS

- Betaine hydrochloride (HCL): 150 mg with each meal (as capsules).
- Digestive enzymes: one to three capsules with each meal.
- Glutamine: 50–150 mg daily.
- Probiotics: one to three capsules or one tablespoon of refrigerated liquid probiotics, up to three times daily before meals; *or* acidophilus: one to three (multi-billion count) capsules before meals.

HERBS

- Cayenne: as directed on label.
- Circumin: as directed on label.
- Fennel: as directed on label.
- Ginger extract (EV EXT 77): 170 mg, one to two times daily (as capsules).
- Licorice root: 450 mg, one to three times daily (as capsules).
- Mint: as directed on label.

CONSIDER / TRY TO

- Acupuncture.
- Detoxification (see TOXICITY on page 280).
- Eat fiber-rich foods.
- Homeopathic remedy for indigestion.

AVOID / WATCH OUT FOR

- Antacids.
- Antibiotics.
- Fried and fatty foods.
- Heavy metals.
- Prescription H2 Blockers, such as Zantac.
- Refined flours and sugars.

Insomnia

Insomnia is the inability to fall asleep or to stay asleep for a sufficient amount of time during regular sleeping hours. It can last for a few nights or more, or it may occur intermittently. It is often caused by anxiety or depression; it can also be a side effect of certain medications, or drinking caffeinated or alcoholic beverages too close to bedtime. Natural remedies can work quite well to ensure a good night's sleep.

SUPPLEMENTS

- Calcium: 500–1,000 mg daily (older women: 1,500–2,000 mg) before bedtime.
- Inositol: 250–500 mg daily.
- Magnesium: 250–500 mg daily before bedtime.
- Melatonin: 1–3 mg, just before bedtime.
- Vitamin B complex: 25–50 mg daily.

HERBS

- Hops: as directed on label.
- Saw palmetto: as directed on label (for men with prostate problems).
- Skullcap: as directed on label.
- St. John's wort (dual action): 300 mg, once or twice daily.
- Valerian: as directed on label.

CONSIDER / TRY TO

- Eat a complex carbohydrate snack a half-hour before bed.
- Exercise regularly.
- Meditation or other stress-relieving techniques.

AVOID / WATCH OUT FOR

- Drugs such as corticosteroids, antidepressants, and cold remedies.
- Excess alcohol, sugar, and caffeine consumption.
- Lots of fluids before bed.
- Muscle tension.

Jaundice

Jaundice is a condition in which excess bile pigment in the blood (known as bilirubin) causes yellowing of the skin and/or eyes. Other symptoms of jaundice can include dark urine. Jaundice may indicate liver disease and other conditions that require medical intervention; however, using the natural remedies listed here with your doctor's approval can help improve the condition.

SUPPLEMENTS

- Complete all-natural multivitamin/mineral complex rich in antioxidants.
- Glutamine: 50–150 mg daily.
- Prebiotic fiber blend: as directed on label.

HERBS

- Dandelion extract: as directed on label.
- Garlic extract: 500 mg, twice daily.
- Grape seed extract: 200 mg daily.
- Green tea extract: 200 mg daily.
- Milk thistle seed extract: 200 mg, three times daily.

CONSIDER / TRY TO

- Eat generous amounts of fresh garlic, oregano, turmeric, artichoke, and coriander daily.
- Increase consumption of fresh fruits and vegetables.

AVOID / WATCH OUT FOR

- Alcohol.
- Caffeine.
- Prescription and over-the-counter drugs unless absolutely necessary.
- Processed foods.
- Processed vegetable oils.
- Smoking.

Jet Lag

JET LAG

The cluster of physical and psychological symptoms associated with travel across time zones is known as jet lag. Characterized by fatigue, difficulty sleeping, mental fogginess, and dehydration, jet lag can spoil the first few days of a vacation or business trip. It's best to prepare yourself prior to travel by getting adequate sleep, drinking plenty of fluids, and staying in as good a shape as possible. There are several natural remedies available to help you readjust to the new time zone so that you can enjoy your trip to the fullest.

SUPPLEMENTS

- Calcium: 500–1,000 mg daily before bedtime (older women: 1,500–2,000 mg).
- Magnesium: 250–500 mg daily before bedtime.
- Melatonin: 1–3 mg, just before bedtime.
- Vitamin B complex: 25–50 mg daily.
- Vitamin C: 500–1,000 mg daily.

HERBS

- Chamomile: as directed on label.
- Hops: as directed on label.
- Skullcap: as directed on label.
- Valerian: as directed on label.

CONSIDER / TRY TO

- Drink six to ten glasses of pure water daily.
- Homeopathic remedy for jet lag.
- Humidifier.

AVOID / WATCH OUT FOR

- Caffeine.
- Drugs.
- Excess alcohol consumption.
- Excess fluids before bed.
- Gaseous foods while flying.
- Stress.

Jock Itch

Jock itch *(Tinea cruris)*, also called groin ringworm, is an itchy, painful fungal infection of the groin and upper and inner thighs. It occurs more frequently in warmer weather and afflicts more men than women. The infection can be quite stubborn—even with diligent application of antifungal products. Fortunately, these products are not your only recourse. Jock itch can be cured, and prevented, by following some commonsense advice and taking a few safe and simple steps.

SUPPLEMENTS

- Caprylic acid: Apply externally twice daily.
- Complete all-natural multivitamin/mineral complex rich in antioxidants.
- Glutamine: 50–150 mg daily.
- MSM: 1,000 mg, three times daily.
- Oregano oil: as directed on label (as capsules).
- Prebiotic fiber blend: as directed on label.

HERBS

- Garlic extract: 500 mg, twice daily.
- Ginger extract (EXT EV 77): 500 mg, one to two times daily (as capsules).
- Olive leaf extract: 500 mg, one to two times daily (as capsules).

CONSIDER / TRY TO

- Drink one or two cups of pau d'arco tea daily.
- Eat generous amounts of fresh garlic daily.
- Increase consumption of fresh vegetables and fish.
- Keep the areas of the affected skin clean and dry.

AVOID / WATCH OUT FOR

- Alcohol and all goods containing yeast.
- Processed foods.
- Smoking and breathing secondhand smoke.
- Wearing tight underwear, athletic supporters and pants.

Kidney Stones

Kidney stones are crystallized stonelike masses of mostly calcium that form in the kidneys. They can range in size from microscopic to an inch or more in diameter. There are many possible causes, including urinary tract infections, heredity, metabolic disorders, and gout. Symptoms may include severe pain, blood in the urine, and a frequent urge to urinate. Drinking plenty of water helps most stones pass out through the urine, and also helps prevent the formation of new ones. There are also a number of other natural steps you can take to remain virtually stone-free.

SUPPLEMENTS

- Calcium: 500–1,000 mg daily (older women: 1,500–2,000 mg).
- Magnesium: 250–500 mg daily.
- Potassium: 99 mg, one to three times daily.
- Vitamin B_6 (pyridoxine): 25–50 mg daily.

HERBS

- Uva ursi: as directed on label.

CONSIDER / TRY TO

- Drink eight to ten glasses of pure water daily.
- Drink orange juice.
- Eat fresh fruits and vegetables, especially lima beans, apricots, bananas, cantaloupe, and potatoes.
- Eat yogurt with live cultures.

AVOID / WATCH OUT FOR

- Large amounts of oxalate-containing foods, such as animal protein.

Legionnaire's Disease

Legionnaire's disease is an acute respiratory
infection caused by the bacterium *Legionella
pneumophila*. This bacterium has been found
in water delivery systems and can survive in
the warm, moist air-conditioning systems of
large buildings, including hospitals. Symptoms
of Legionnaire's disease include fever, chills,
muscle aches, headache, tiredness, loss of
appetite, and, occasionally, diarrhea. Left
untreated, Legionnaire's disease can cause
pneumonia, so it is essential to start treatment
early. Fortunately, there are a number of natural
remedies that have been proven effective in
helping to fight this disease.

SUPPLEMENTS

- Acidophilus capsule or refrigerated liquid form taken along with prescribed antibiotics.
- Complete all-natural multivitamin/mineral complex rich in antioxidants.
- Vitamin C: 500 to 1,000 mg, twice daily.

HERBS

- Astragalus: 500 mg, twice daily.
- Garlic: 500 mg, twice daily.

CONSIDER / TRY TO

- Eat more fruits and vegetables, especially darker ones.
- Eat whole foods.
- Eat yogurt with live cultures.

AVOID / WATCH OUT FOR

- Smoking.
- Stress.
- Sugar and processed carbohydrates.

Lice

LICE

Head lice are tiny parasitic insects that favor hairy parts of the human body, usually the head. Lice infestation causes intense itchiness and may lead to secondary infections, such as dermatitis. The condition is easily transmitted by personal contact and through the use of personal items such as brushes, combs, hats, and the like. Although it is thought of as a difficult-to-treat condition, lice and their eggs (known as nits) can be exterminated with the proper steps and diligent care.

SUPPLEMENTS

- Complete all-natural multivitamin/mineral complex rich in antioxidants.
- MSM (with vitamin C complex): 1,000 mg daily.

HERBS

- Garlic extract: 500 mg, twice daily.

CONSIDER / TRY TO

- Apply aloe vera gel to irritated skin, including the scalp.
- Boil brushes, combs, curlers, and other hair products.
- Keep the scalp clean and dry.
- Wash clothes and linens frequently with hot water and dry them on the hottest setting.

AVOID / WATCH OUT FOR

- Contact with infected people.
- Sharing hats, hairbrushes, combs, clothing, bed linens, or pillows with others.

Lung Cancer

Lung cancer is the most common cancer in both men and women. The overwhelming majority of lung cancer cases are caused by cigarette smoking. The symptoms of lung cancer vary to some degree, but the main symptom is almost always a persistent cough. The best prevention for lung cancer is to quit smoking, but if you are a longtime smoker, it is highly recommended that you get regular screenings and take nutritional supplements. See also CANCER PREVENTION.

LUNG CANCER

SUPPLEMENTS

- Carotenoids: 10,000–20,000 IU daily.
- Selenium: 100–200 mcg daily.
- Vitamin E: 400–500 IU daily.

HERBS

- Grape seed/green tea complex: 100 mg of each, twice daily.

CONSIDER / TRY TO

- Eat raw vegetables and fruits.

AVOID / WATCH OUT FOR

- Automobile fumes.
- Secondhand smoke.
- Smoking.

Lung Cancer

185

Lupus

Systemic lupus erythematosus (SLE)—generally known as lupus—is an autoimmune disease, meaning that the immune system cannot distinguish between self and non-self. Symptoms vary from person to person and range in severity from mild to debilitating, and include rash, sun sensitivity, sores, and inflammation of tendons, joints, and other tissues and organs. Taking nutritional supplements and other positive steps can help control inflammation, relieve pain, restore vitality, and reduce the chance and frequency of flare-ups.

SUPPLEMENTS

- Complete all-natural multivitamin/mineral complex rich in antioxidants.
- DHEA: 100–200 mg, first thing in the morning (check with practitioner for exact dose).
- Glucosamine sulfate potassium: 1,000–1,500 mg daily.
- MSM: 1,000 mg, three times daily.

HERBS

- Evening primrose oil: 500 mg, two to three times daily (as capsules).
- Ginger (EXT EV 77): 170 mg, one to three times daily (as capsules).

CONSIDER / TRY TO

- Drink herbal teas such as ginger, licorice, red clover, and milk thistle daily.
- Eat more foods rich in omega-3 fatty acids.
- Eat more raw fruits and vegetables.
- Eat soy foods daily.
- Reduce stress.

AVOID / WATCH OUT FOR

- Alcohol.
- All commercially processed oils.
- Caffeine.
- Stress.

Lyme Disease

Lyme disease is caused by the spiral-shaped bacteria *Borrelia burgdorferi*, which is usually spread by deer ticks. It generally presents itself as a large red spot (resembling a "bull's eye") on the body. Other symptoms, including chills, fever, fatigue, and muscle aches, commonly follow. Arthritis may also develop, even years after the initial infection. While prevention is always the best medicine, the symptoms of Lyme disease respond well to natural remedies.

SUPPLEMENTS

- Complete all-natural multivitamin/mineral complex rich in antioxidants.
- Glucosamine sulfate potassium: 1,000–1,500 mg daily.
- Glutamine: 50–150 mg daily.
- MSM: 1,000 mg, three times daily.

HERBS

- Echinacea: 100–500 mg daily for two weeks.
- Feverfew extract: 300 mg, twice daily.
- Garlic extract: 500 mg, twice daily.
- Turmeric: 500 mg, three times daily (as capsules).
- White willow bark: 325 mg, twice daily.

CONSIDER / TRY TO

- Apply hot/cold packs (alternate) to inflamed joints.
- Drink herbal teas such as ginger, red clover, milk thistle, and peppermint.
- Eat more foods rich in omega-3 fatty acids.
- Eat plain, unsweetened yogurt daily.

AVOID / WATCH OUT FOR

- Alcohol.
- Caffeine.
- Deadly nightshades such as peppers, white potatoes, and tomatoes.
- Foods that contain artificial colors, flavors, and preservatives.
- Prescription and over-the-counter drugs unless absolutely necessary.
- Smoking.
- Wheat and dairy products (except yogurt).

Macular Degeneration

Macular degeneration is a degenerative eye disorder that results in a gradual loss of vision generally in both eyes. This disorder tends to be hereditary and usually occurs later in life. It doesn't normally cause complete blindness—peripheral vision is usually unaffected. It's not possible to reverse this disorder; however, further degeneration can be slowed with nutritional supplementation.

SUPPLEMENTS

- Carotenoids: 10,000–20,000 IU daily.
- Complete all-natural multivitamin/mineral complex rich in antioxidants.
- Lutein: 6–20 mg daily.
- Selenium: 100–200 mcg daily.
- Vitamin C: 500–1,000 mg daily.
- Zinc: 15 mg of elemental zinc (read label), once or twice daily.

HERBS

- Ginkgo biloba extract: 60 mg, one to three times daily.
- Grape seed/green tea complex: 100 mg of each, twice daily.

CONSIDER / TRY TO

- Eat more peas, oysters, and lean meats.

AVOID / WATCH OUT FOR

- High-fat foods.
- Low-fiber foods.
- Smoking.
- Sugar.

Memory Loss

Forgetfulness is often attributed to the normal effects of aging; however, there's no reason an otherwise healthy adult can't retain a sharp memory well into old age. While memory loss can be a symptom of Alzheimer's disease, senile dementia, and other neurodegenerative disorders, it can also simply be a result of inadequate nutrition, lack of sleep, a side effect of certain medications, or other easily remedied problems. Restoring and maintaining a good memory is possible by supplementing the diet with natural memory-promoting nutrients and by making simple lifestyle changes.
See also ALZHEIMER'S DISEASE; SENILE DEMENTIA.

MEMORY LOSS

SUPPLEMENTS

- Choline: 500–1,000 mg daily.
- DMAE: 75 mg, once or twice daily.
- Folic acid: 400–800 mcg daily.
- L-Carnitine: 50–500 mg daily.
- Pantothenic acid (vitamin B_5): 30–100 mg daily.
- Phosphatidyl serine: 15 mg, once or twice daily.
- Pregnenolone: 10 mg daily.
- Vitamin B_1 (thiamin): 50–500 mg daily.
- Vitamin B_{12}: 100–1,000 mcg daily.
- Zinc: 15 mg of elemental zinc (read label), once or twice daily.

HERBS

- Bacopa extract: 100 mg daily.
- Club moss (Huperzine A): as directed on label.
- Fo-ti: as directed on label.
- Ginkgo biloba extract: 60 mg, one to three times daily.
- Gotu kola: as directed on label.
- Schizandra: as directed on label.
- Siberian ginseng root: as directed on label.
- Vinpocetine: as directed on label.

CONSIDER / TRY TO

- Exercise regularly.
- Get enough sleep (at least seven to eight hours).
- Yoga.

AVOID / WATCH OUT FOR

- Alcohol.
- Drugs that interfere with brain function.
- High blood pressure.
- Poor diet.
- Stress.

Menopausal Symptoms

Menopause is the period in a woman's life when menstruation stops. It doesn't occur overnight, of course; it can take anywhere from one to two years. Problems associated with menopause can include hot flashes, dryness of the vaginal walls, night sweats, irritability, loss of bone calcium, and depression. Fortunately, there are many natural remedies a woman can use to ease the troublesome symptoms of menopause so that she can pass through this stage of her life in relative comfort. See also VAGINAL DRYNESS.

SUPPLEMENTS

- Calcium: 500–1,000 mg daily (older women: 1,500–2,000 mg).
- Magnesium: 250–500 mg daily.
- NAC (N-acetylcysteine): 1,500 mg with meals daily.
- Natural progesterone cream: use as directed on label.
- Soy isoflavonoids: 40–60 mg daily.
- Vitamin B_6 (pyridoxine): 25–50 mg daily.
- Vitamin C: 500–1,000 mg daily.

HERBS

- Anise: as directed on label.
- Dong quai: as directed on label.
- Fennel: as directed on label.
- Ginseng: as directed on label.
- Licorice root: 450 mg, one to three times daily (as capsules).
- Red clover: as directed on label.
- Vitex (chasteberry): as directed on label.

CONSIDER / TRY TO

- Eat more fresh fruits and vegetables.
- Eat soy foods.
- Exercise regularly.
- Lose weight if necessary.
- Natural estrogen cream for vaginal dryness.

AVOID / WATCH OUT FOR

- Excess weight.
- Junk food.
- Lack of exercise.
- Stress.
- Synthetic hormones (HRT).

Migraines

Migraines are recurrent painful headaches, sometimes severe, that commonly affect only one side of the head, but sometimes affect both. They are caused by the restriction and dilation of blood vessels in the head. An attack may last several hours or even days. People who get migraines commonly turn to prescription and over-the-counter medications for relief. However, natural remedies can be just as effective, are safer, and can even reduce the frequency of attacks. See also HEADACHES.

SUPPLEMENTS

- Calcium: 500–1,000 mg daily (older women: 1,500–2,000 mg).
- Magnesium: 250–500 mg daily.
- Niacin (vitamin B_3): 50–1,000 mg daily, in divided doses.
- Vitamin B complex: 25–50 mg daily.

HERBS

- Feverfew: as directed on label.
- Ginkgo biloba extract: 60 mg, one to three times daily.
- Peppermint: as directed on label.
- St. John's wort (dual action): 300 mg, once or twice daily.
- White willow bark: 500–1,000 mg, two to three times daily (as capsules).

CONSIDER / TRY TO

- Relaxation.
- Use a headband.

AVOID / WATCH OUT FOR

- Alcohol.
- Excess stress.
- Stressor foods, including fat, caffeine, alcohol, sugar, and salt.
- Tobacco.

Mononucleosis

Mononucleosis (sometimes called the "kissing disease" by adolescents) is caused by infection with the Epstein-Barr virus. It is passed from person to person through infected saliva and mucus. Symptoms generally include fever, swollen glands, sore throat, loss of appetite, and fatigue and may last for several weeks. Bed rest and drinking plenty of fluids are the usual recommendations. In addition to these steps, natural remedies can boost the immune system and bring relief of symptoms sooner.

SUPPLEMENTS

- Complete all-natural multivitamin/mineral complex rich in antioxidants.
- Glutamine: 50–150 mg daily.
- Vitamin C complex: 1,000 mg, twice daily.
- Zinc: 15 mg of elemental zinc daily.

HERBS

- Echinacea and American feverfew adaptogen: one dropper, three times daily for one month.

CONSIDER / TRY TO

- Drink eight to ten glasses of pure water daily.
- Eat more fresh fruits and vegetables.

AVOID / WATCH OUT FOR

- Processed foods containing artificial flavorings, colors, or preservatives.

Multiple Sclerosis

Multiple sclerosis (MS) is a disorder of the central nervous system, which includes the brain and spinal cord. This condition occurs when the immune system goes haywire and attacks the body's nerve coverings (myellin). Symptoms differ with each person and may include double vision, mood swings, numbness, tingling, and coordination problems. There are many natural ways to cope with the symptoms, including getting regular exercise and stretching to control coordination and range of motion.

SUPPLEMENTS

- Complete all-natural multivitamin/mineral complex rich in antioxidants.
- Coenzyme Q_{10}: 60 mg, twice daily.
- Glutamine: 50–150 mg daily.
- MSM: 1,000 mg, three times daily.
- Threonine: 6 grams daily.

HERBS

- Evening primrose oil: 500 mg, twice daily.
- Garlic extract: 500 mg, twice daily.
- Grape seed extract: 200 mg daily.
- Green tea extract: 200 mg daily.

CONSIDER / TRY TO

- Drink eight to ten glasses of pure water daily.
- Test for food and environmental allergies.
- Test for toxic levels of heavy metals in blood.

AVOID / WATCH OUT FOR

- Alcohol.
- Caffeine.
- Dairy products (except plain, unsweetened yogurt).
- Exposure to extreme hot or cold temperatures.
- Foods rich in trans fatty acids.
- Processed foods containing artificial flavorings, colors, or preservatives.
- Refined carbohydrates, especially sugar and white flour.
- Smoking and breathing secondhand smoke.

Muscle Cramps

Muscle cramps—a painful contraction of a muscle or group of muscles—are usually harmless and last only a few minutes. While a muscle cramp now and then is virtually inevitable, it is possible to take preventive steps, such as stretching before and after exercise and other physical tasks, to reduce the frequency of cramps. Certain nutritional supplements also help the muscles expand and contract with more fluidity, thereby reducing the likelihood of cramping even further.

MUSCLE CRAMPS

SUPPLEMENTS

- Calcium: 1,000 mg, twice daily or at bedtime (older women: 1,500–2,000 mg).
- Complete all-natural multivitamin/mineral complex rich in antioxidants.
- Magnesium: 400 mg, twice daily or at bedtime.
- Malic acid: 1,200–2,400 mg daily.
- Potassium: 99 mg daily.
- Vitamin E complex (with tocotrienols): 400 IU, two to three times daily.

HERBS

- Garlic extract: 500 mg, twice daily.
- Horse chestnut (standardized extract with Aescin): 50 mg, twice daily (as tablets).

CONSIDER / TRY TO

- Drink eight to ten glasses of pure water daily.
- Eat more whole foods, such as fresh fruits and vegetables.
- Hot bath before bed with mineral salts added.
- Massage muscles that are prone to cramping.

AVOID / WATCH OUT FOR

- Prescription drugs that can cause cramping, such as diuretics, estrogens, and lithium.
- Smoking.

Muscle Pull

A pulled muscle can be very painful, but the pain is usually not long-lasting. It can occur from overextension or overuse during exercise or even during regular daily activities, such as lifting a child or a heavy household item. To prevent muscle pulls, it is very important to stretch often to maintain muscle flexibility and to warm up properly before workouts. Pushing yourself past your limits should be avoided. Certain steps can help prevent muscle pulls, while others relieve the pain once the pull has occurred. See also SPRAINS AND STRAINS.

SUPPLEMENTS

- Vitamin B_6 (pyridoxine): 25–50 mg daily.
- Vitamin B_{12}: 100–1,000 mcg daily.
- Vitamin C: 500–1,000 mg daily with 500 mg of bioflavonoids daily.

HERBS

- Arnica ointment: apply topically as directed on label.
- Eucalyptus ointment: apply topically as directed on label.
- Grape seed extract (PCOs): 100 mg, one to three times daily.
- White willow bark: 500–1,000 mg, two to three times daily (as capsules).

CONSIDER / TRY TO

- Drink six ounces of water every fifteen to twenty minutes while exercising.
- Stretch before workouts.

AVOID / WATCH OUT FOR

- Cola drinks.
- Fried foods.
- Refined flour.
- Strenuous exercise.
- White sugar.

Nausea

Nausea is the uncomfortable feeling in the stomach that usually precedes vomiting, but it can also occur alone. There are a number of causes, including motion sickness, certain drugs, flu, and even psychological problems, to name just a few. When a person is nauseous, immediate relief of the unpleasant feeling is highly desired. Vomiting usually brings relief— at least for a little while. Natural remedies work to settle the stomach and bypass the need to vomit.

SUPPLEMENTS

- Glutamine: 50–150 mg daily.
- Vitamin B complex: 25–50 mg daily.
- Vitamin B_6 (pyridoxine): 25–50 mg daily.
- Vitamin C: 500–1,000 mg daily.
- Vitamin K: 100 mcg daily.

HERBS

- Basil: as directed on label.
- Chamomile: as directed on label.
- Ginger extract (EV EXT 77): 170 mg, one to two times daily (as capsules).
- Licorice root: 450 mg, one to three times daily (as capsules).
- Peppermint tea: drink as needed.

CONSIDER / TRY TO

- Acupressure.
- Detoxification (see TOXICITY on page 280).

AVOID / WATCH OUT FOR

- Greasy foods.
- Overeating.
- Prescription drugs.

Night Blindness

Night blindness is a condition in which a person
has difficulty seeing at night or in dim light but
has no problem seeing during daylight hours.
The most common cause of night blindness is
a vitamin A deficiency. Anyone suffering from
this disorder should have a complete eye
examination, as night blindness may point to
the development of a more serious disorder
such as retinitis pigmentosa. In cases where
night blindness is caused by a lack of vitamin A,
supplements of this vitamin, as well as other
natural remedies, can improve the condition
considerably.

SUPPLEMENTS

- Alpha-lipoic acid: 50 mg daily.
- Coenzyme Q_{10}: 60 mg, twice daily.
- Complete all-natural multivitamin/mineral complex rich in antioxidants and 10,000 IU of beta-carotene.
- MSM: 1,000 mg, three times daily.
- Selenium: 200 mcg daily.
- Vitamin A: 5,000 IU daily.
- Zinc: 15 mg of elemental zinc daily.

HERBS

- Bilberry extract: 60 mg, twice daily.
- Ginkgo biloba: 60 mg, twice daily.

CONSIDER / TRY TO

- Eat a high-protein diet.
- Eat plenty of fresh fruits and vegetables.
- Exercise regularly.
- Have your eyes checked.
- Maintain a healthy body weight.
- Reduce stress.

AVOID / WATCH OUT FOR

- Alcohol.
- Excessive exposure to sun.
- Processed carbohydrates such as sugar and white flour.
- Smoking.
- Stress.

Nosebleeds

Nosebleeds can occur for a variety of reasons, from something as simple as a blow to the nose to more serious conditions, such as leukemia. In most cases, a simple nosebleed—in which the blood comes from a broken blood vessel inside the nose—can be controlled by applying pressure to the sides of the nose. A gauze packing may help control the loss of blood when the flow cannot otherwise be controlled. Frequent nosebleeds should be reported to a doctor, but occasional nosebleeds respond well and occur less frequently when natural therapies are applied.

SUPPLEMENTS

- Complete all-natural multivitamin/mineral complex rich in antioxidants.
- Vitamin C: 1,000 mg, three times daily.
- Vitamin K: 80 mcg daily.

HERBS

- Bilberry extract: 60 mg, twice daily.
- Grape seed extract: 200 mg daily.
- Green tea extract: 200 mg daily.
- Horse chestnut extract: 500 mg, three times daily.

CONSIDER / TRY TO

- Apply liquid vitamin E to nostrils.
- Increase consumption of dark green vegetables high in vitamin K.
- Run a humidifier to moisten dry air, especially during the winter.
- Sniff a small amount of powdered yarrow.

AVOID / WATCH OUT FOR

- Alcohol.
- Certain drugs, such as corticosteroids, warfarin (coumadin), aspirin, antibiotics, and oral contraceptives.
- Commercial nasal sprays.
- Smoking and breathing secondhand smoke.

Oral Cancer

Oral cancer predominantly affects those over the age of forty, although it can affect certain young people who abuse chewing tobacco. The most common cause of oral cancer, like lung cancer, is cigarette smoking. Early signs of the disease include a lump or mass on the inside of the mouth or a white or red patch of tissue in the mouth that refuses to heal. As with lung cancer, the best prevention for oral cancer is to quit smoking. See also CANCER PREVENTION.

SUPPLEMENTS

- Beta-carotene: 10,000–20,000 IU daily.
- Multiple antioxidant formula: as directed on label.
- Spirulina: 1,000 mg, one to three times daily.
- Vitamin E: 400–500 IU daily.

HERBS

- Green tea extract: 100 mg, twice daily, or drink one cup of tea daily.

CONSIDER / TRY TO

- Eat darkly colored fresh fruits and vegetables.

AVOID / WATCH OUT FOR

- Excessive alcohol consumption.
- Tobacco (all forms).

Osteomalacia

Osteomalacia is a condition that affects adults in which the bones become soft due to a loss of calcium from the skeleton. Bones become flexible and deformities can result. One common cause of osteomalacia is a lack of vitamin D. People with kidney or liver disorders are also at risk for osteomalacia because they may be unable to convert vitamin D into usable form. In addition to other natural remedies, taking daily vitamin D and calcium supplements may help.

SUPPLEMENTS

- Boron: 2 mg daily.
- Calcium: 1,000 mg daily (older women: 1,500–2,000 mg).
- Complete all-natural multivitamin/mineral complex rich in antioxidants.
- Magnesium: 400 mg daily.
- MSM: 1,000 mg, three times daily.
- Vitamin D: 400 IU daily.

HERBS

- Garlic extract: 500 mg, twice daily.
- Glucosamine sulfate potassium: 1,000–1,500 mg daily.
- Silica: 70 mg daily.

CONSIDER / TRY TO

- Eat more foods rich in omega-3 fatty acids, such as salmon, tuna, herring, and cod.
- Eat more vitamin D rich foods, including salmon, tuna, cod liver oil, eggs, mushrooms, sunflower seeds, and cheese.
- Increase consumption of snow peas, broccoli, spinach, kale, beets, turnip greens, almonds, figs, beans, whole grains, wheat bran, bananas, apricots, and other rich sources of calcium and magnesium.

AVOID / WATCH OUT FOR

- Alcohol.
- Caffeine and cola drinks.
- Foods rich in trans fatty acids.
- High-protein diets.
- Stress.

Osteoporosis

Osteoporosis is a thinning of the bones that can eventually lead to fractures and deformity. It is usually the result of a progressive decrease in calcium reabsorption into the bones and is most common in postmenopausal women and the elderly. Common symptoms of osteoporosis include painful backaches and frequent fractures. Osteoporosis, however, is not a necessary evil of old age. It can often be treated effectively or even be prevented with a complete regimen of natural remedies.

SUPPLEMENTS

- Acidophilus: one to three (multi-billion count) capsules before meals.
- Boron: 2 mg daily.
- Calcium: 500–1,000 mg daily (older women: 1,500–2,000 mg).
- Omega-3 fatty acids: 50 mg, one to three times daily (as fish oil capsules).
- Magnesium: 250–500 mg daily.
- Manganese: 9 mg daily.
- Vitamin D: 200–800 IU daily.
- Zinc: 15 mg of elemental zinc (read label), once or twice daily.

HERBS

- Butcher's broom: as directed on label.
- Garlic: 500 mg daily.
- Grape seed extract (PCOs): 100 mg, one to three times daily.
- Horsetail: as directed on label.
- Licorice root: 450 mg, one to three times daily (as capsules).

CONSIDER / TRY TO

- Eat soy products.
- Gentle weight-bearing exercises.
- Natural progesterone cream.

AVOID / WATCH OUT FOR

- Excess caffeinated sodas (leaches calcium from bone).
- Excess protein (leaches calcium from bone).
- Prescription drugs, such as cortisones and corticosteroids.

Overweight/Obesity

A large percentage of Americans are overweight or obese. Generally speaking, when more calories are consumed than are used by the body, weight gain results. People often turn to the latest fad diet to rid themselves of extra pounds. These diets, however, are seldom successful in the long run. Losing excess weight and keeping it off requires persistence and patience, but it can be achieved by implementing healthy eating habits and getting regular exercise. Exercise can be as simple as a daily brisk walk or laps in the pool. Also, taking certain nutritional and herbal supplements may help melt away the pounds more quickly.

SUPPLEMENTS

- Complete all-natural multivitamin/mineral complex rich in antioxidants.
- Glutamine: 50–150 mg daily.
- L-Carnitine: 1,000–2,000 mg daily.
- MSM: 1,000 mg twice daily.
- Vanadium: 100 mcg daily.
- Zinc: 15 mg of elemental zinc daily.

HERBS

- Banana leaf extract: 45 mg daily.
- Gymnema sylvestre: 400 mg daily.
- Phaseolus vulgaris: 45 mg daily.

CONSIDER / TRY TO

- Drink eight to ten glasses of pure water daily.
- Drink several cups of green tea daily.
- Eat a high-protein diet, low in processed carbohydrates, sugar, and salt.
- Eat more fiber.
- Eat more foods rich in omega-3 fatty acids, such as deep water fish.
- Exercise daily for thirty minutes.

AVOID / WATCH OUT FOR

- Alcohol.
- Foods rich in trans fatty acids.
- Skipping meals, especially breakfast.
- Snacks and junk food.

Pain

Everyone has experienced some kind of pain
at one time or another. Pain is defined as an
unpleasant sensation signaling that the body
is damaged or threatened by an injury. Pain
can result from a wide range of causes, from
lacerations, fractures, and bruises to diseases
such as cancer, arthritis, and AIDS. Most people
turn to some type of analgesic (pain reliever)
such as aspirin, codeine, or morphine to treat
their pain. However, it can often be treated as
effectively with the use of a variety of natural
methods, which do not have the potentially
serious side effects of drugs.

SUPPLEMENTS

- Choline: 500–1,000 mg daily.
- Digestive enzymes: one to three times daily with each meal (as capsules).
- DLPA (dl-phenylalanine): 375–750 mg, every four hours for discomfort (as capsules).
- Glucosamine hydrochlorida: 600–1,200 mg daily.
- Vitamin B_1 (thiamin): 50–500 mg daily.
- Vitamin B complex: 25–50 mg daily.

HERBS

- Aloe vera gel (cuts, wounds, and burns): apply topically as directed on label.
- Arnica gel (bruising and swelling): apply topically as directed on label.
- Calendula ointment or gel: apply topically as directed on label.
- Capsaicin: as directed on label.
- Feverfew (headache): as directed on label.
- Ginger extract (EV EXT 77): 170 mg, one to two times daily (as capsules).
- White willow bark: 500–1,000 mg, two to three times daily (as capsules).

CONSIDER / TRY TO

- Acupuncture/acupressure.
- Alternate between hot and cold packs.
- Exercise regularly.
- Meditation, tai chi, and/or yoga.

AVOID / WATCH OUT FOR

- Coffee.
- Improper lifting (back pain).
- NSAIDs (nonsteroidal anti-inflammatory drugs).
- Stress.

Panic Attacks/Disorder

A panic attack is a bout of extreme anxiety accompanied by physical symptoms such as dizziness, shaking, sweating, difficulty breathing, chest pain, and a racing heart. A person suffering from a panic attack often feels as if he or she is going to die. When these attacks occur often and unexpectedly, the condition is known as panic disorder. Antidepressants and anxiety drugs are often prescribed to reduce the frequency of attacks, but there is no need to resort to prescription drugs. There are many natural remedies that can reduce the frequency of attacks, as well as their severity.

SUPPLEMENTS

- Calcium: 1,000 mg daily (older women: 1,500–2,000 mg).
- Complete all-natural multivitamin/mineral complex rich in antioxidants.
- Glutamine: 50–150 mg daily.
- L-Tyrosine: 500 mg, three times daily.
- Magnesium: 400 mg daily.

HERBS

- Ginkgo biloba: 60 mg, twice daily.
- Skullcap: 500 mg, one to three times daily (as capsules).
- St. John's wort (dual action): 300 mg, twice daily.
- Valerian: 500 mg, one to three times at bedtime (as capsules).

CONSIDER / TRY TO

- Exercise daily for thirty minutes.
- Increase consumption of apricots, avocados, bananas, brown rice, salmon, garlic, leafy green vegetables, raw nuts and seeds, and plain, unsweetened yogurt.
- Relax.

AVOID / WATCH OUT FOR

- Alcohol.
- Caffeine.
- Refined carbohydrates, sugar, soft drinks, and chocolate.

Periodontitis

Untreated gingivitis (see page 134) eventually
leads to periodontitis—a main cause of tooth
loss in adults. It occurs when an overgrowth
of bacteria decay the supporting structures of
the teeth, namely the roots and bone. Unlike
gingivitis, periodontitis cannot be corrected
simply with good oral hygiene. Professional
intervention by a periodontist is required, but
recovery and continued oral health can be
achieved with some natural care.

PERIODONTITIS

SUPPLEMENTS

- Coenzyme Q_{10}: 60 mg, three times daily.
- Complete all-natural multivitamin/mineral complex rich in antioxidants.
- Glutamine: 50–150 mg daily.
- MSM: 1,000 mg, three times daily.
- Vitamin C complex: 500 mg, three times daily.

HERBS

- Echinacea: 100–500 mg daily for no more than two weeks.
- Garlic extract: 500 mg, twice daily.
- Ginger extract (EXT EV 77): 500 mg, two to three times daily (as capsules).
- Golden seal: 1,000 mg, three times daily for one week only.
- Grape seed extract: 200 mg daily.
- Green tea extract: 200 mg daily.

CONSIDER / TRY TO

- Drink several cups of green tea daily.
- Eat generous amounts of fresh garlic and onions daily.
- Reduce stress.
- Test for toxic levels of heavy metals in the blood.

AVOID / WATCH OUT FOR

- Alcohol.
- Smoking and breathing secondhand smoke.
- Stress.
- Teeth grinding.

Premenstrual Syndrome (PMS)

PMS is a condition in which a variety of symptoms, including nervousness, irritability, depression, headaches, tissue swelling, and breast tenderness, may occur up to fourteen days before a woman starts her period. It usually disappears soon after the period begins. Although women often turn to over-the-counter drugs for relief, there are a number of natural remedies that can be used to alleviate many of the troublesome symptoms of PMS.

PREMENSTRUAL SYNDROME (PMS)

SUPPLEMENTS

- Calcium: 500–1,000 mg daily (older women: 1,500–2,000 mg).
- Complete all-natural multivitamin/mineral complex rich in antioxidants.
- Essential fatty acids: 250 mg, one to three times daily (as capsules).
- Iron (organic): 10–15 mg of essential iron daily.
- Magnesium: 250–500 mg daily.
- Manganese: 9 mg daily.
- Soy isoflavonoids: 40–60 mg daily.
- Vitamin A: 5,000–10,000 IU daily.
- Vitamin B_6 (pyridoxine): 25–50 mg daily.
- Vitamin C: 500–1,000 mg daily.
- Vitamin E: 400–500 IU daily.
- Zinc: 15 mg of elemental zinc (read label), once or twice daily.

HERBS

- Dong quai: as directed on label.
- Ginkgo biloba extract: 60 mg, one to three times daily.
- Licorice root: 450 mg, one to three times daily (as capsules).
- Milk thistle (silymarin): 140 mg, one to three times daily.
- Vitex (chasteberry): as directed on label.
- Wild yam: as directed on label.

CONSIDER / TRY TO

- Eat dandelion greens and other leafy green vegetables.
- Eat more protein and fewer fats.
- Exercise regularly and do gentle weightlifting.

AVOID / WATCH OUT FOR

- Birth control pills/synthetic hormones.
- Dairy products, refined carbohydrates, and sugar.
- Estrogen dominance.
- Excess colas or other caffeinated soda and coffee.

Prostate, Enlarged

The prostate is a small gland nestled around the urethra, the duct that drains the bladder. In many men over age forty-five, the gland tends to gradually grow larger. If the gland grows too large, it can begin to squeeze the urethra, making urination difficult. Those who suffer from an enlarged prostate often feel the need to urinate more frequently and feel that their urinations are incomplete. Treatment of this condition usually focuses on shrinking the prostate, which can often be accomplished using a variety of natural remedies. See also PROSTATE CANCER.

SUPPLEMENTS

- Glycine: 50 mg, one to three times daily.
- Glutamine: 50–150 mg daily.
- Selenium: 100–200 mcg daily.
- Vitamin B_6 (pyridoxine): 25–50 mg daily.
- Vitamin C: 500–1,000 mg daily.
- Vitamin E: 400–500 IU daily.
- Zinc: 15 mg of elemental zinc (read label), once or twice daily.

HERBS

- Nettles: as directed on label.
- Pygeum: as directed on label.
- Saw palmetto: as directed on label.

CONSIDER / TRY TO

- Drink six to eight glasses of pure water daily.
- Eat pumpkin seeds, a good source of zinc.
- Eat soy products, cold-water fish, fresh fruits and vegetables, and yogurt with live cultures.

AVOID / WATCH OUT FOR

- Excess alcohol consumption.
- Fatty foods and junk foods.
- Hydrogenated oils.
- Stress.
- Sugar.

Prostate Cancer

Cancer of the prostate is extremely common in elderly men, though its exact cause isn't known. It tends to grow very slowly over a period of many years and eventually gives symptoms similar to those of an enlarged prostate, if any. The best prevention for prostate cancer is early detection, and regular prostate screenings for men over age forty-five are highly recommended. See also CANCER PREVENTION; PROSTATE, ENLARGED.

SUPPLEMENTS

- Complete all-natural multivitamin/mineral complex rich in antioxidants.
- Lutein: 6–20 mg daily.
- Lycopene: 6–10 mg daily.
- Soy isoflavonoids: 40–60 mg daily.

HERBS

- No herbs apply.

CONSIDER / TRY TO

- Eat soybeans and tofu.

AVOID / WATCH OUT FOR

- Diet high in saturated fats.

Psoriasis/Eczema

Psoriasis and eczema are both very common diseases of the skin that are accompanied by scaling, inflammation, itchiness, and redness. Although both are rarely serious, they are often very uncomfortable and can make those who suffer from them self-conscious. With the use of natural methods, however, psoriasis and eczema can often be treated and controlled very effectively.

SUPPLEMENTS

- Omega-3 fatty acids: 50 mg, one to three times daily (as fish oil capsules).
- Selenium: 100–200 mcg daily.
- Vitamin A: 5,000–10,000 IU daily.
- Vitamin D: 200–800 IU daily.

HERBS

- Aloe vera gel: apply topically as directed on label.
- Capsaicin: as directed on label.
- Yellow dock: as directed on label.

CONSIDER / TRY TO

- Lose weight if necessary.

AVOID / WATCH OUT FOR

- Excess alcohol consumption.
- High-fat foods.
- Stress.

Raynaud's Disease

Raynaud's disease is a condition in which the fingers and toes become pale, splotchy, or bluish as a result of arterial spasms in the extremities—usually upon exposure to cold. Uncomfortable numbness, tingling, and burning sensations in the hands and feet are common complaints. Warming the extremities provides relief, but treating the disorder from the inside out with natural remedies can help reduce the severity of the condition.

RAYNAUD'S DISEASE

SUPPLEMENTS

- Calcium: 1,000 mg daily (older women: 1,500–2,000 mg).
- Coenzyme Q_{10}: 60 mg daily.
- Complete all-natural multivitamin/mineral complex rich in antioxidants.
- Magnesium: 400 mg daily.
- MSM: 1,000 mg, three times daily.

HERBS

- Garlic extract: 500 mg, twice daily.
- Ginger extract: 500 mg, twice daily.
- Ginkgo biloba: 60 mg, twice daily.

CONSIDER / TRY TO

- Drink eight to ten glasses of pure water daily.
- Exercise regularly.
- Increase consumption of whole foods, foods rich in omega-3 fatty acids, and fresh garlic and ginger.
- Reduce stress.
- Wear shoes that fit comfortably.

AVOID / WATCH OUT FOR

- Alcohol.
- Caffeine.
- Certain prescription drugs, such as calcium channel blockers, betablockers, ergotamines, oral contraceptives, diet pills, and decongestants.
- Fried foods.
- Processed carbohydrates, sugar and white flour.
- Smoking.

Rectal Cancer

Rectal cancer is very closely linked to colon cancer, and the diseases together are often referred to as colorectal cancer. Diet and heredity both seem to play major roles in increasing the risk of developing this disease. Common symptoms of rectal cancer include blood in the stool, change in bowel habits, and frequent vomiting. Certain dietary changes, as well as the use of nutritional supplements, may help in the prevention of rectal cancer. See also CANCER PREVENTION; COLON CANCER.

SUPPLEMENTS

- Calcium: 500–1,000 mg daily (older women: 1,500–2,000 mg).
- Folic acid: 400–800 mcg daily.

HERBS

- Psyllium: as directed on label.

CONSIDER / TRY TO

- Eat nuts, fruits, and vegetables.
- Eat oat fiber.
- Eat soy foods, including soy protein shakes.

AVOID / WATCH OUT FOR

- Low-fiber foods.
- Saturated fats.

Restless Leg Syndrome

RESTLESS LEG SYNDROME

Also known as Ekbom syndrome, restless leg syndrome is a condition in which an irritating sense of uneasiness and itching, often accompanied by twitching and pain, is felt in the calves of the legs when sitting or lying. The only relief is walking or moving the legs, which unfortunately sometimes leads to insomnia. Natural remedies, however, can often help to alleviate the symptoms of this condition.

RESTLESS LEG SYNDROME

SUPPLEMENTS

- Calcium: 500–1,000 mg daily (older women: 1,500–2,000 mg).
- Vitamin E: 400–500 IU daily.

HERBS

- Butcher's broom: as directed on label.
- Ginkgo biloba extract: 60 mg, one to three times daily.
- Horse chestnut: as directed on label.

CONSIDER / TRY TO

- Exercise regularly.

AVOID / WATCH OUT FOR

- Sitting in one position for a long time.

Ringworm

Ringworm is a highly contagious fungal infection that presents itself as discolored ring-shaped patches of skin on the body. When it infects the feet, it is known as athlete's foot (see page 32) and when it infects the groin, it is known as jock itch (see page 176). Inadequately treated ringworm can be quite persistent and difficult to control. Topical or oral antifungal medicine is conventionally used to treat the condition, but often without lasting success. Natural remedies make it possible to first get ringworm under control and then eliminated entirely.

SUPPLEMENTS

- Caprylic acid: as directed on label.
- Complete all-natural multivitamin/mineral complex rich in antioxidants.
- Digestive enzymes: once with each meal (as capsules).
- MSM: 1,000 mg, three times daily.
- MSM lotion: apply topically to affected areas up to three times daily.

HERBS

- Berberine extract: 250 mg, three times daily (after meals).
- Garlic extract: 500 mg, twice daily.
- Ginger extract: 500 mg, twice daily.
- Grape seed extract: 200 mg daily.
- Green tea extract: 200 mg daily.
- Olive leaf extract: 500 mg, twice daily.

CONSIDER / TRY TO

- Check your pets for signs of ringworm. Patches of hair loss are a dead give-away.
- Keep areas of the skin affected clean and dry.
- Oregano oil and tea tree oil applied directly to affected area.

AVOID / WATCH OUT FOR

- All forms of sugar, white flour, and refined carbohydrates.
- Smoking and breathing secondhand smoke.
- Wearing tight, sweaty shoes.

Rosacea

Rosacea, sometimes incorrectly called adult acne, is a chronic inflammatory condition of the face—most often the central area. Telltale signs of this malady include persistent redness, prominent blood vessels, and pimple-like pustules. Although the cause of this condition is unknown and there is no cure for rosacea, the things that trigger a flare-up—such as alcohol consumption, unprotected sun exposure, and extremes of temperature—are relatively easy to avoid. Antibiotics and topical solutions are often prescribed to control the condition, but this can be accomplished with the use of natural remedies and careful avoidance of triggers.

SUPPLEMENTS

- Complete all-natural multivitamin/mineral complex rich in antioxidants.
- Evening primrose oil: 500 mg, three times daily.
- Flaxseed oil: 500 mg, twice daily.
- Zinc: 15 mg of elemental zinc daily.

HERBS

- Dandelion extract: 500 mg, one to three times daily (as capsules).
- Grape seed extract: 200 mg daily.
- Green tea extract: 200 mg daily.
- Silica: 30 mg daily.

CONSIDER / TRY TO

- Drink eight to ten glasses of pure water daily.
- Eat generous amounts of garlic and onions.
- Eat plain, unsweetened yogurt daily.
- Keep face clean to prevent infections.
- Reduce stress.

AVOID / WATCH OUT FOR

- Alcohol.
- Caffeine.
- Excessive sun exposure.
- Extreme temperatures, saunas, and freezing cold.
- Fried or spicy food.
- Hot beverages.

Scabies

The parasitic skin infection known as scabies is caused by *Sarcoptes scabiei*, a barely visible mite that burrows under the skin. Symptoms include intense itching, especially at night. The burrows are visible to the naked eye and look like small wavy lines on the skin's surface. Scabies spread through skin-to-skin contact, but quickly die on clothing and bedding. Conventional treatments often irritate the skin, while natural remedies eliminate the condition without irritating side effects.

SUPPLEMENTS

- Complete all-natural multivitamin/mineral complex rich in antioxidants.
- MSM: 1,000 mg, three times daily.
- Zinc: 15 mg of elemental zinc daily.

HERBS

- Garlic extract: 500 mg, twice daily.
- Rhubarb, black walnut, pau d'arco or wormwood extracts: as directed on label.

CONSIDER / TRY TO

- Drink eight to ten glasses of pure water daily.
- Eat generous amounts of fresh garlic and onions daily.
- Keep areas of the affected skin clean and dry.

AVOID / WATCH OUT FOR

- Do not share bed linens with anyone who is infected.
- Limit consumption of fruit and fruit juice, vinegar, aged cheese, wheat, potatoes, tomatoes, carbohydrates, sugar, white flour, and other processed foods.
- Skin-to-skin contact.

Seasonal Affective Disorder (SAD)

Seasonal affective disorder (SAD) is an intense feeling of sadness beginning from the fall and lasting through the winter. It is possible that SAD is caused by an extended duration of the secretion of the hormone melatonin, which normally occurs at night. Symptoms of SAD include lethargy, oversleeping, overeating, and a decreased interest in otherwise pleasant activities. Nutritional supplements, regular exercise, and natural remedies can help reduce symptoms naturally.

SEASONAL AFFECTIVE DISORDER (SAD)

SUPPLEMENTS

- Complete all-natural multivitamin/mineral complex rich in antioxidants.
- L-Tyrosine: 3,000 mg at night on an empty stomach.
- Vitamin B complex: 50 mg, twice daily.

HERBS

- Ginseng extract: 500 mg, two to three times daily (American ginseng capsules preferred).
- St. John's wort (dual action): 300 mg, two to three times daily.

CONSIDER / TRY TO

- Eat a high-protein diet.
- Eat foods rich in tryptophan, such as turkey, chicken, avocado, walnuts, bananas, soy products, seeds, nuts, whole grains, brown rice, and legumes.
- Light therapy.
- Reduce stress.
- Spend more time outdoors.

AVOID / WATCH OUT FOR

- Alcohol.
- Caffeine and chocolate.
- Foods containing artificial flavorings, colors, or preservatives.
- Processed foods, especially sugar, white flour, and other refined carbohydrates.

Senile Dementia

Senile dementia is defined as the loss of intellectual faculties, often associated with behavioral deterioration, beginning for the first time in old age. Most people who suffer from this disease have impaired memory, judgment, and learning ability, and often their personalities deteriorate. The most common causes of senile dementia are Alzheimer's disease and strokes. With the aid of natural therapies, the symptoms of senile dementia can often be alleviated and sometimes even be prevented. See also ALZHEIMER'S DISEASE; MEMORY LOSS.

SUPPLEMENTS

- Coenzyme Q_{10}: 60 mg, one to three times daily.
- DHEA: 25 mg daily for women over forty;
  50 mg daily for men over forty.
- Folic acid: 400–800 mcg daily.
- NADH: 10 mg on an empty stomach daily.
- Natural progesterone cream: use as directed
  on label (for women).
- Niacin: 50–1,000 mg daily, in divided doses.
- Vitamin B_{12}: 100–1,000 mcg daily.
- Vitamin C: 500–1,000 mg daily.
- Vitamin E: 400–500 IU daily.
- Zinc: 15 mg of elemental zinc (read label),
  once or twice daily.

HERBS

- Bacopa extract: 100 mg daily.
- Club moss (Huperzine A): as directed on label.
- Ginkgo biloba extract: 60 mg, one to three
  times daily.

CONSIDER / TRY TO

- Drink pure water in excess of eight glasses daily.
- Eat high-fiber foods and more protein.

AVOID / WATCH OUT FOR

- Aluminum foil and cookware.
- Environmental toxins, such as pesticides.
- Fumes from solvents, paints, and glues.
- Prescription drugs.
- Vitamin B_{12} deficiency.

Shingles

Shingles infection causes fluid-filled blisters accompanied by moments of intense shooting pain. Pain may linger even after the infection has cleared. Although it can affect anyone at any age, it usually occurs in those aged fifty and over. It is caused by the same virus that causes chickenpox (see page 78). After the initial infection, this virus remains dormant in the nerves and may never cause further problems. However, lowered immune function and other factors may reactivate the virus. While shingles must run its course, nutritional supplements along with adequate rest can speed the process along.

SUPPLEMENTS

- Complete all-natural multivitamin/mineral complex rich in antioxidants.
- L-Lysine: 500 mg, three times daily (between meals).
- MSM: 1,000 mg, three times daily.

HERBS

- Astragalus: 400 mg, twice daily.
- Cayenne extract: 500 mg, one to three times daily (as capsules).
- Elderberry extract: Four tablespoons daily (two tablespoons for children).
- Garlic extract: 500 mg, twice daily.
- Olive leaf extract: 500 mg, twice daily.

CONSIDER / TRY TO

- Eat generous amounts of fresh garlic, onions, ginger, and shiitake and reishi mushrooms daily.
- Keep affected areas of the skin clean and dry.
- Take cool baths.
- Wear loose-fitting clothes.

AVOID / WATCH OUT FOR

- Alcohol.
- Caffeine.
- Drugs.

Sinusitis

Inflammation of the sinuses (the hollow cavities in the bones around the nose) is known as sinusitis. It is usually due to allergy or to a bacterial, viral, or fungal infection. It can be either a short-lived or an ongoing condition. Symptoms of sinusitis include pain below the eyes and over the cheeks, headache, and toothache. Antibiotics are often prescribed, and sometimes, over-the-counter remedies are used. However, natural remedies work just as well and do not have the associated side effects of common medications. See also ALLERGIES TO DUST, MOLD, AND DANDER; HAY FEVER; TOOTHACHE.

SINUSITIS

SUPPLEMENTS

- Coenzyme Q_{10}: 60 mg, one to three times daily.
- MSM: 1,000 mg, one to three times daily.
- Vitamin A: 5,000–10,000 IU daily.
- Vitamin B complex: 25–50 mg daily.
- Vitamin C: 500–1,000 mg daily.
- Zinc: 15 mg of elemental zinc (read label), once or twice daily.

HERBS

- Echinacea: as directed on label.
- Garlic: 500 mg daily.
- Goldenseal: as directed on label.

CONSIDER / TRY TO

- Drink hot liquids.
- Drink pure water in excess of eight glasses daily.
- Eat more raw fruits and vegetables.
- Nasal irrigation with water, salt, and baking soda solution.

AVOID / WATCH OUT FOR

- Allergenic foods.
- Dairy products.
- Dust and pollen.
- Forceful nose blowing.
- Irritant fumes and smoke.
- Overuse of decongestants.

Skin Cancer

Skin cancer is the most common type of cancer, but most types are curable. The more common forms of skin cancer usually develop on sun-exposed areas. People who have had a lot of sun exposure, particularly those with fair complexions, are most likely to develop this type of cancer. A telltale sign of skin cancer is the emergence of a new growth or enlarging mole on the surface of the skin, which should be brought to a doctor's attention as soon as possible. See also CANCER PREVENTION.

SUPPLEMENTS

- Carotenoids: 10,000–20,000 IU daily.
- Multiple antioxidant formula: as directed on label.
- Vitamin C: 500–1,000 mg daily.

HERBS

- No herbs apply.

CONSIDER / TRY TO

- Eat more vegetables, especially Swiss chard, pumpkin, cabbage, Brussels sprouts, and broccoli.
- Use sun block with SPF 15 or higher.

AVOID / WATCH OUT FOR

- Diet high in saturated fat.
- Overexposure to sun.

Skin Irritations

There are many different kinds of skin irritations, which can be treated in any number of ways. Acne, rashes, dermatitis, and eczema are all considered irritations of the skin. They are usually marked by a redness or an inflammation on the surface of the skin. Drugstores stock countless products that are aimed at alleviating these irritations, but there are a number of natural therapies that are equally effective in not only treating these irritations, but also preventing further ones from developing.

SUPPLEMENTS

- MSM: 1,000 mg, one to three times daily.
- Omega-3 fatty acids: 50 mg, one to three times daily (as fish oil capsules).
- Selenium: 100–200 mcg daily.
- Vitamin A: 5,000–10,000 IU daily.
- Vitamin D: 200–800 IU daily.

HERBS

- Aloe vera gel: apply topically as directed on label.
- Capsaicin: as directed on label.
- Gotu kola: as directed on label.

CONSIDER / TRY TO

- Drink six to ten glasses of pure water daily.

AVOID / WATCH OUT FOR

- Excessive alcohol consumption.
- High-fat foods.
- Sugar.

Smoking Dependency

Anyone who smokes knows how difficult it is to quit for good. They also know how dangerous cigarette smoking is to themselves and to those who breathe in their secondhand smoke. From gum and patches to inhalers and pills, smoking remedies are filling drugstore shelves. While they may work for a select few, the majority of smokers need a better way. Many do not realize that help can come in the form of the nutritional and herbal supplements. With a little willpower and some help from nature, there is a way to quit smoking, once and for all.

SUPPLEMENTS

- Calcium: 500 mg, three times daily (older women: 1,500–2,000 mg).
- Coenzyme Q_{10}: 60 mg, three times daily.
- Magnesium: 200 mg, three times daily.
- MSM: 1,000 mg, three times daily.
- Vitamin B complex: 50 mg, twice daily (with food).
- Vitamin C complex: 500 mg, three times daily.

HERBS

- Cayenne: 500 mg, two to three times daily (as capsules).
- Milk thistle: 140 mg, two to three times daily (as capsules).
- Slippery elm lozenges: dissolve in mouth up to three times daily.
- St. John's wort (dual action): 300 mg, two to three times daily (after stopping smoking).

CONSIDER / TRY TO

- Chew on raw, unsalted sunflower seeds (shelled) whenever you have a craving for a cigarette.
- Drink eight to ten glasses of pure water daily.
- Eat more onions, garlic, leafy green vegetables, nuts, and seeds.
- Quit smoking.

AVOID / WATCH OUT FOR

- Caffeine.
- Peanuts, animal protein, junk food, processed refined foods, saturated fats, salt, sugar, and white flour.
- Stress.

Sore Throat

SORE THROAT

A sore throat is common to anyone who has had a bad cold or flu, or yelled too much at a sporting event. It is defined as a pain at the back of the mouth, which is commonly due to a bacterial or viral infection of the tonsils, larynx, or the pharynx, or to an overuse of the vocal cords. A sore throat can also be an indicator of something more serious, such as strep throat or mononucleosis. While many people turn to antibiotics, medicated lozenges, and other medicines to treat their sore throats, many natural therapies are just as effective.

SUPPLEMENTS

- Acidophilus: one to three (multi-billion count) capsules before each meal.
- Vitamin A: 5,000–10,000 IU daily.
- Vitamin C: 500–1,000 mg daily.
- Zinc lozenges: one lozenge dissolved in mouth, two to three times daily.

HERBS

- Echinacea: as directed on label.
- Garlic: 500 mg daily.
- Goldenseal: as directed on label.
- Slippery elm: as directed on label.

CONSIDER / TRY TO

- Drink plenty of liquids.
- Gargle with echinacea/goldenseal water or saltwater.
- Swallow one tablespoon of honey mixed with lemon juice.

AVOID / WATCH OUT FOR

- Dust and pollen.
- Gum or tooth infections.
- Heavy coughing.
- Smoke and fumes.
- Very hot food and drinks.

Sprains and Strains

Sprains and strains, while often painful, are almost always treatable. A sprain is an injury to a ligament that is usually caused by a sudden overstretching. A strain is the excessive stretching of a muscle, resulting in pain and swelling of the muscle. While the passage of time and reduced use of the affected ligament or muscle is the best remedy, recovery from sprains and strains can be speeded up with the help of a regimen of natural remedies. See also MUSCLE PULL.

SUPPLEMENTS

- Calcium: 500–1,000 mg daily (older women: 1,500–2,000 mg).
- Digestive enzymes: one to three capsules with each meal.
- Magnesium: 250–500 mg daily.
- Vitamin B complex: 25–50 mg daily.
- Vitamin C: 500–1,000 mg daily with 500 mg of bioflavonoids daily.
- Zinc: 15 mg of elemental zinc (read label), once or twice daily.

HERBS

- Aloe vera gel: apply topically as directed on label.
- Arnica gel: apply topically as directed on label.
- Calendula ointment or gel: apply topically as directed on label.

CONSIDER / TRY TO

- Alternate between heat packs and ice packs.
- Eat extra protein.
- Take hot baths with Epsom salts and baking soda.

AVOID / WATCH OUT FOR

- Excess consumption of aspirin, ibuprofen, and acetaminophen.
- Overexercising.

Stomach Cancer

Stomach cancer usually affects older people. The symptoms of this type of cancer are similar to those of a peptic ulcer, namely burning, aching, soreness, and an empty feeling. While its causes have not been confirmed, dietary factors are thought to play a key role. Thus, a healthy diet and a regimen of natural supplements can be crucial in preventing this disease. See also CANCER PREVENTION.

SUPPLEMENTS

- Multiple antioxidant formula: as directed on label.
- Vitamin C: 500–1,000 mg daily.

HERBS

- Garlic: 500 mg daily.
- Grape seed/green tea complex: 100 mg of each, twice daily.

CONSIDER / TRY TO

- Eat onions, leeks, chives, garlic, and shallots.

AVOID / WATCH OUT FOR

- Nitrites and nitrates, commonly found in luncheon meats, hot dogs, sausages, jerky, and bacon.

Stress

Stress is any factor that puts a strain on the body. It can be physical or psychological in nature. Stress can result from injury, disease, infection, overwork, financial worries, changes in the environment, relationship conflicts, and even too much of a "good thing." When the body is stressed by any one factor, it is more susceptible to other stressors. When you are stressed-out, try to reduce, treat, or eliminate the stressor from your life, and turn to natural remedies to build up your resistance.

SUPPLEMENTS

- Calcium: 500–1,000 mg daily (older women: 1,500–2,000 mg).
- DHEA: 25 mg daily for women over forty; 50 mg daily for men over forty.
- Magnesium: 250–500 mg daily.
- Melatonin: 1–3 mg, just before bedtime.
- Vitamin B complex: 25–50 mg daily.

HERBS

- Chamomile: as directed on label.
- Siberian ginseng: as directed on label.
- St. John's wort (dual action): 300 mg, once or twice daily.
- Valerian: as directed on label.

CONSIDER / TRY TO

- Exercise regularly.
- Massage.

AVOID / WATCH OUT FOR

- Stressor foods, including fat, caffeine, alcohol, sugar, and salt.
- Tobacco.

Stroke

A stroke (apoplexy) is a sudden attack of weakness affecting one side of the body, a consequence of an interruption of the flow of blood to the brain. Early symptoms include slurred speech, becoming dizzy or confused, and blurred or lost vision. Strokes are caused by high blood pressure, diabetes, high cholesterol, and smoking. A program of natural remedies can be very effective in preventing the onset of a stroke, and can also help with recovery. See also CARDIOVASCULAR DISEASE.

SUPPLEMENTS

- Calcium: 500–1,000 mg daily (older women: 1,500–2,000 mg).
- Carotenoids: 10,000–20,000 IU daily.
- Omega-3 fatty acids: 50 mg, one to three times daily (as fish oil capsules).
- Potassium: 99 mg, one to three times daily.
- Selenium: 100–200 mcg daily.
- Vitamin A: 5,000–10,000 IU daily.
- Vitamin D: 200–800 IU daily.
- Vitamin E: 400–500 IU daily.

HERBS

- Alfalfa: as directed on label.
- Ginger extract (EV EXT 77): 170 mg, one to two times daily (as capsules).
- Ginkgo biloba extract: 60 mg, one to three times daily.
- Rutin: 50 mg, one to three times daily.
- Tarragon oil: as directed on label.
- Turmeric: as directed on label.

CONSIDER / TRY TO

- Eat more cruciferous vegetables.
- Exercise regularly.

AVOID / WATCH OUT FOR

- Alcohol consumption.
- Excess weight.
- High blood pressure.
- Salt and sugar.
- Smoking.
- Stress.

Sunburn

Sunburn results from an overexposure to ultraviolet (UV) rays. Depending on the amount of sun exposure and type of skin pigment a person has, the skin becomes red, swollen, and painful. Later, blisters may form, and the skin may peel. Staying out of strong, direct sunlight is the most obvious and effective way to prevent sunburn. When exposed to the sun, the use of sunscreen is highly recommended. Natural remedies can help speed recovery and reduce the chance of permanent damage.

SUPPLEMENTS

- Potassium: 99 mg, one to three times daily.
- Vitamin C: 500–1,000 mg daily.
- Vitamin E: 400–500 IU daily.

HERBS

- Aloe vera gel: apply topically as directed on label.
- Arnica lotion: apply topically as directed on label.
- Calendula ointment: apply topically as directed on label.
- Chamomile tea: apply topically in compresses.

CONSIDER / TRY TO

- Drink lots of fluids.
- Rub MSM lotion on affected skin.
- Wear sunglasses, sun hat, and loose clothing.

AVOID / WATCH OUT FOR

- Excessive exposure to the sun.
- Retin-A and tetracycline (otherwise, when taking these drugs, avoid excessive exposure to the sun).

Surgery

If you are facing surgery, chances are you want to do all you can to make sure you are in tip-top condition. After surgery, you will want to recover as soon as possible. Certain nutritional supplements and herbs can help bring your body to peak condition before surgery and can help return your body to a healthy state afterward. Be sure to let your surgeon know that you are taking supplements. Find out how long before the scheduled surgery you should stop taking them and when would be a good time to resume using them.

SUPPLEMENTS

- Coenzyme Q_{10}: 60 mg, one to three times daily.
- Vitamin A: 5,000–10,000 IU daily.
- Vitamin C: 500–1,000 mg daily.
- Vitamin E: 400–500 IU daily.
- Zinc: 15 mg of elemental zinc (read label), once or twice daily.

HERBS

- Ginseng tea: drink one cup daily.
- Grape seed/green tea complex: 100 mg of each twice daily.
- Licorice root: 450 mg, one to three times daily (as capsules).
- Milk thistle (silymarin): 140 mg, one to three times daily (as capsules).
- St. John's wort (dual action) (for anxiety): 300 mg, once or twice daily.
- White willow bark: 500–1,000 mg, two to three times daily (as capsules).
- *See caution under "Avoid / Watch Out For" below.*

CONSIDER / TRY TO

- Drink lots of fluids after surgery.
- Eat more fiber-rich foods.

AVOID / WATCH OUT FOR

- Alcohol for forty-eight hours before and after surgery.
- Herbs for forty-eight hours before surgery; check with your surgeon before resuming.
- Highly processed foods.
- Refined sugar and food additives.

Taste Loss

Taste loss is rarely ever a life-threatening condition, but it certainly takes away from the enjoyment of sitting down to a delicious meal. The senses of taste and smell are closely linked. If you cannot smell your food, as in the case of a stuffed nose, your sense of taste will be diminished. This is usually a temporary condition. Loss of taste can also result from smoking, as a side effect of prescription medications, or from burns to the taste buds. Natural remedies, especially supplementing with zinc, can restore taste to make eating the enjoyable experience it should be.

SUPPLEMENTS

- Complete all-natural multivitamin/mineral complex rich in antioxidants.
- Zinc: 15 mg of elemental zinc (read label), once or twice daily.

HERBS

- No herbs apply.

CONSIDER / TRY TO

- Saltwater nasal drops.

Tinnitus

Tinnitus, the sensation of ringing or buzzing in the ears, is a relatively common problem that ranges in severity. Although the exact cause is unknown, it can be a complication of almost any disorder that affects the ears, such as ear infections and hearing loss. It may also occur as a result of head trauma, Méniére's disease, and a number of other conditions. Tinnitus can be quite bothersome and, in rare cases, debilitating, but fortunately, there are steps that can be taken to reduce the severity of the condition or perhaps eliminate it entirely, depending on the cause.

SUPPLEMENTS

- Calcium: 500 mg at bedtime.
- Coenzyme Q_{10}: 60 mg, twice daily.
- Complete all-natural multivitamin/mineral complex rich in antioxidants.
- Glutamine: 50–150 mg daily.
- Inositol hexanicotinate (no-flush niacin): 200 mg, three times daily.
- Magnesium: 200 mg at bedtime.

HERBS

- Ginkgo biloba: 60 mg, three times daily.

CONSIDER / TRY TO

- Clean ears regularly to avoid ear wax buildup.
- Eat generous amounts of fresh onions and garlic.
- Eat a high-protein diet.
- Reduce stress.

AVOID / WATCH OUT FOR

- Alcohol.
- Caffeine.
- Exposure to loud noises. Use earplugs when necessary.
- Recreational drugs.
- Refined carbohydrates.
- Smoking.

Toothache

Anyone who has had a toothache knows just how painful and annoying they can be. A toothache may result from a cavity, an abscess, inflammation of the gum around the root of the tooth, or sinus inflammation. In cases of very painful toothaches, immediate attention by a dentist is very important. For milder toothaches and to prevent them from occurring, a number of natural remedies can be highly effective. However, even in the case of mild toothaches, make an appointment to see your dentist. See also SINUSITIS.

SUPPLEMENTS

- Calcium: 500–1,000 mg daily (older women: 1,500–2,000 mg).
- Coenzyme Q_{10}: 60 mg, one to three times daily.
- Folic acid: 400–800 mcg daily.
- Vitamin C: 500–1,000 mg daily with 500 mg of bioflavonoids daily.
- Vitamin D: 200–800 IU daily.

HERBS

- Evening primrose oil: 500–1,000 mg daily (as capsules).
- Green tea extract: 100 mg tablets, twice daily, or drink one to two cups of tea daily.
- Oil of cloves: apply to affected area with a toothpick.

CONSIDER / TRY TO

- Bite chili peppers.
- Brush carefully.
- Use a gum stimulator.

AVOID / WATCH OUT FOR

- Dried fruits.
- High-carbohydrate foods.
- Potato chips.
- Sipping sugared beverages.

Toxicity

There are many toxins, or poisons, in our environment—bacteria, fumes, heavy metals, drugs, and so on—that can all contribute to an overall toxic condition. This toxic condition can contribute to, or aggravate, many other ailments discussed in this book. A good detoxification program, such as the one suggested on the facing page, can not only help you feel better overall, but can also help clear up stubborn symptoms attributed to other causes.

SUPPLEMENTS

- Fiber: 6–12 grams daily.
- Glutamine: 50–150 mg daily.
- MSM: 1,000 mg, one to three times daily.
- Multi–trace mineral formula: as directed on label.

HERBS

- Burdock root: as directed on label.
- Cascara sagrada: as directed on label.
- Dandelion: as directed on label.
- Echinacea: as directed on label.
- Goldenseal: as directed on label.
- Licorice root: 450 mg, one to three times daily (as capsules).
- Milk thistle (silymarin): 140 mg, one to three times daily (as capsules).
- Oregon grape root: as directed on label.
- Parsley: as directed on label.
- Uva ursi: as directed on label.
- Yellow dock: as directed on label.

CONSIDER / TRY TO

- A professional high colonic enema.
- Drink six to eight glasses of pure water daily.
- Eat more fiber-rich foods.
- Sit in a sauna once daily.

AVOID / WATCH OUT FOR

- Environmental toxins/pollution.
- Excess alcohol consumption.
- Junk food.

Ulcer, Peptic

A peptic ulcer is a well-defined round sore where the lining of the stomach has been eaten away by stomach acid and digestive juices. It usually develops when the defense mechanisms protecting the stomach from acid break down. Ulcer symptoms—gnawing, soreness, and burning in the stomach—tend to occur when the stomach is empty and often come and go as the day wears on. While most people turn to antacids and other such medicines to relieve them of ulcers, many natural therapies can be just as effective and are usually safer. See also DIGESTIVE DISORDERS.

SUPPLEMENTS

- Betaine hydrochloride (HCL): 150 mg, with each meal (as capsules).
- Digestive enzymes: one to three capsules with each meal.
- Glutamine: 50–150 mg daily.
- Pectin: 500–1,500 mg daily.
- Vitamin E: 400–500 IU daily.

HERBS

- Aloe vera juice: one tablespoon twice daily.
- Cabbage juice: one tablespoon two to three times daily.
- Cayenne: as directed on label.
- Licorice root: 450 mg, one to three times daily (as capsules).
- Papaya: one to three tablets after a meal or eat the fruit after a large meal.

CONSIDER / TRY TO

- Eat yogurt with live cultures.

AVOID / WATCH OUT FOR

- Animal fats.
- Caffeine, alcohol, and soda.
- Fried foods.
- NSAIDs (nonsteroidal anti-inflammatory drugs).
- Salt and strong spices.

Urinary Tract Infection

The kidneys, bladder, ureters, and urethra comprise the urinary tract. Urinary tract infections are commonly caused by bacteria, but may also be caused by fungi, viruses, or parasites. A common infection of the urinary tract is urethritis—infection of the urethra. Symptoms include pain during urination and a frequent urge to urinate. This condition is often treated with antibiotics; however, it is possible to treat it naturally and prevent it from occurring by incorporating simple steps into your daily routine. See also CYSTITIS.

URINARY TRACT INFECTION

SUPPLEMENTS

- Magnesium: 250–500 mg daily.
- Vitamin A: 5,000–10,000 IU daily.
- Vitamin B$_6$ (pyridoxine): 25–50 mg daily.
- Vitamin C: 500–1,000 mg daily.

HERBS

- Cranberry juice extract: as directed on label.
- Marshmallow root: as directed on label.
- Oregon grape root: as directed on label.
- Uva ursi: as directed on label.

CONSIDER / TRY TO

- Acupuncture.
- Always wipe front to back.
- Drink six to eight glasses of pure water daily.
- Drink two 8-ounce glasses of unsweetened cranberry juice daily.
- Homeopathic bladder infection remedy.
- Take a sitz bath.
- Urinate when you feel the urge and immediately after intercourse.

AVOID / WATCH OUT FOR

- Holding urine.
- Tight-fitting clothing.
- Wiping back to front.

Vaginal Dryness

One of the primary symptoms of menopause, vaginal dryness leads to irritation, inflammation, itching, and tenderness of the vagina. Continued dryness sometimes leads to yeast infections and vaginitis. Vaginal dryness is not something that should be simply accepted as an inevitable consequence of menopause. There are quite a few natural methods that can be used to help alleviate the problem. See also MENOPAUSAL SYMPTOMS.

VAGINAL DRYNESS

SUPPLEMENTS

- None apply.

HERBS

- Dong quai: as directed on label.
- Vitex (chasteberry): as directed on label.

CONSIDER / TRY TO

- Eat more protein.
- Natural progesterone cream (if that does not work, try a small amount of natural estrogen cream).

AVOID / WATCH OUT FOR

- Excess weight.
- Overexercising.
- Stress.
- Synthetic hormones (hormone replacement therapy; HRT).

Vaginal Yeast Infection

A yeast infection (candidiasis) is a very common infection of the vagina that causes discharge, itching, and swelling. It is caused by a fungus called *Candida*, which lives in the body all the time but occasionally gets out of control. People with diabetes and pregnant women are particularly prone to this infection. It is not serious and can often be relieved with the help of natural remedies. See also CANDIDIASIS.

SUPPLEMENTS

- Acidophilus: one to three (multi-billion count) capsules before each meal.
- Caprylic acid supplement: one to three times daily.
- Garlic: 500 mg daily.
- MSM: 1,000 mg, one to three times daily.
- Shiitake mushroom extract: as directed on label.

HERBS

- Barberry: as directed on label.
- Chamomile: as directed on label.
- Cinnamon: as directed on label.
- Dandelion: as directed on label.
- Echinacea: as directed on label.
- Licorice root: 450 mg, one to three times daily (as capsules).
- Pau d'arco: as directed on label.

CONSIDER / TRY TO

- Boric acid solution douche.
- Eat raw garlic.
- Eat shiitake mushrooms.
- Tea tree oil douche.

AVOID / WATCH OUT FOR

- Simple carbohydrates.
- Yeast-containing foods.

Varicose Veins

Varicose veins, which usually occur in the legs, are bluish, swollen, stretched veins that can often be seen bulging through the skin. This condition sometimes causes discomfort and aching in the legs, especially when it is first beginning to develop. Thought to be due in part to heredity, varicose veins cannot be reversed. Surgery to remove as many of the veins as possible is sometimes undertaken. However, natural steps can be taken to improve the appearance of the veins, reduce the associated discomfort, and possibly reduce the chances of more developing.

VARICOSE VEINS

SUPPLEMENTS

- Bioflavonoids: 500 mg daily to strengthen capillaries.
- Vitamin E: 400–500 IU daily.

HERBS

- Buckthorn: as directed on label.
- Butcher's broom: as directed on label.
- Cascara sagrada: as directed on label.
- Ginkgo biloba extract: 60 mg, one to three times daily.
- Gotu kola: as directed on label.

CONSIDER / TRY TO

- Detoxification (see TOXICITY on page 280).
- Eat more fiber for bowel movements.
- Eat more fruits and vegetables.
- Exercise regularly, including stretching.
- Yoga.

AVOID / WATCH OUT FOR

- High-fat diet.
- Hot, spicy foods.
- Sitting for long periods.
- Straining during bowel movements.

Vertigo

People with vertigo have the uncomfortable sensation that either they or the objects around them are spinning or moving. This is often accompanied by a loss of balance and feelings of nausea. Vertigo, which can last from several hours to a few days, has several causes, the most common of which is motion sickness. Motion sickness itself results from heightened sensitivity of the inner ear to movement. Natural remedies can help prevent a bout with vertigo as well as help reduce the unsettling feeling once it's occurred.

Vertigo

SUPPLEMENTS

- Calcium: 500–1,000 mg daily (older women: 1,500–2,000 mg).
- Vitamin B$_6$ (pyridoxine): 25–50 mg daily.

HERBS

- Ginger root extract: as directed on label.
- Ginkgo biloba extract: 60 mg, one to three times daily.

CONSIDER / TRY TO

- Acupuncture.
- Low-salt diet.

AVOID / WATCH OUT FOR

- Amusement-park rides.
- Boating.
- Glass elevators in high-rise buildings.

Vision Problems

As people age, visual acuity, or clarity of vision, tends to decrease, and vision becomes blurry. Many consider this an inevitable effect of advancing age. Middle-aged people often discover that their eyesight "isn't what it used to be." However, your eyesight doesn't "have to go" just because you're getting older. In addition to regularly seeing an ophthalmologist, taking natural steps now can protect your vision later in life. See also CATARACTS.

SUPPLEMENTS

- N-acetylcysteine: 1,500 mg with meals.
- Selenium: 100–200 mcg daily.
- Vitamin A: 5,000–10,000 IU daily.
- Vitamin C: 500–1,000 mg daily.
- Vitamin E: 400–500 IU daily.

HERBS

- Bilberry extract: as directed on label.
- Evening primrose oil: 500–1,000 mg daily (as capsules).
- Ginkgo biloba extract: 60 mg, one to three times daily.
- Grape seed extract (PCOs): 100 mg, one to three times daily.
- Quercetin: 400 mg before eating, one to three times daily.

CONSIDER / TRY TO

- Eat fish rich in omega-3 fatty acids.
- Eat green, orange, and yellow vegetables.

AVOID / WATCH OUT FOR

- Excess sugar consumption.
- Hydrogenated oils.
- Prescription drugs.

Vitiligo (Leukoderma)

Vitiligo, also known as leukoderma, is a type
of skin-pigmentation disorder characterized by
smooth white patches of skin on various parts
of the body. It occurs when the melanocytes
(skin cells) stop producing the skin pigment
melanin. The reason this occurs is still under
investigation. The condition itself is benign
and does not cause any physical discomfort,
but it often causes affected people to feel
self-conscious. There currently is no standard
medical treatment to reverse the condition;
however, natural remedies have proven
themselves very helpful.

VITILIGO (LEUKODERMA)

SUPPLEMENTS

- Complete all-natural multivitamin/mineral complex rich in antioxidants.
- Glutamine: 50–150 mg daily.
- MSM: 1,000 mg, three times daily.
- Zinc: 30 mg of elemental zinc daily.

HERBS

- Khellin extract: 100–160 mg daily.
- Picrorrhiza: as directed on label.

CONSIDER / TRY TO

- Apply walnut juice to affected areas as a natural cosmetic to darken white spots.
- Drink eight to ten glasses of pure water daily.
- Exercise regularly.
- Keep affected areas of the skin clean and dry.
- Reduce stress.

AVOID / WATCH OUT FOR

- Commercial cosmetics.
- Excessive sunlight.
- Processed and fried foods.
- Smoke.

Warts

Warts—those unsightly growths on the skin—
are caused by infection with the human
papillomavirus. Most warts are harmless, but
can easily spread from one area of the body to
another. While most warts disappear on their
own within a few years, some do persist or
recur. There's no reason to wait it out or to
resort to chemicals or freezing to rid yourself of
warts when there are simple, natural, effective
steps you can take to clear up this unsightly
viral infection.

SUPPLEMENTS

- Complete all-natural multivitamin/mineral complex rich in antioxidants.
- L-cysteine: 500 mg, twice daily.
- MSM: 1,000 mg, three times daily.
- Vitamin C complex: 1,000 mg, three times daily.

HERBS

- Garlic extract: 500 mg, twice daily.
- Olive leaf extract: 500 mg, twice daily.

CONSIDER / TRY TO

- Apply aloe vera gel directly on warts two to three times daily.
- Apply fresh, crushed garlic directly on warts and secure with a bandage for twenty-four hours.

AVOID / WATCH OUT FOR

- Alcohol.
- Caffeine.
- Refined carbohydrates and sugar.
- Smoking.
- Stress.

Wounds

A wound is defined as a break in the structure of an organ or tissue caused by an external agent. Put simply, if you've ever been bruised, grazed, cut, punctured, or burned, you've received a wound. Wounds are treated in a variety of ways, depending on severity and type. There are many natural remedies that can be very effective in helping to heal wounds more quickly.

SUPPLEMENTS

- Bromelain: as directed on label.
- Vitamin C: 500–1,000 mg daily.
- Vitamin E: 400–500 IU daily.
- Zinc: 15 mg of elemental zinc (read label), once or twice daily.

HERBS

- Aloe vera gel: apply topically as directed on label.
- Calendula ointment or gel: apply topically as directed on label.
- Comfrey tea: apply topically.

CONSIDER / TRY TO

- Vitamin E cream.
- Wash with antibacterial soap and water.

AVOID / WATCH OUT FOR

- Aspirin and other blood-thinners.

Wrinkles

Wrinkles are usually thought of as one the first signs of aging. As we age, our skin becomes less firm, resulting in some creases and lines that are ultimately unavoidable. The number of wrinkles we develop and the severity of them, however, can be controlled. The best thing that can be done to protect your skin from wrinkles is to avoid excessive exposure to sunlight as much as possible. Beyond that, there are a number of natural methods and remedies that can be used to both help protect and restore vitality to your skin.

SUPPLEMENTS

- Complete all-natural multivitamin/mineral complex rich in antioxidants.
- DHEA: 25 mg daily for women over forty; 50 mg daily for men over forty.
- Nucleic Acids (RNA and DNA): 100–300 mg daily.
- SOD (Superoxidedismutase): 125 mcg daily.
- Vitamin C: 500–1,000 mg daily.
- Vitamin E: 400–500 IU daily.

HERBS

- Wild yam: as directed on label.

CONSIDER / TRY TO

- Drink six to ten glasses of pure water daily.
- Eat fresh fruits and vegetables.
- Get enough sleep (at least seven to eight hours).
- Lose weight if necessary.

AVOID / WATCH OUT FOR

- Excessive sun exposure.

Therapies

ACUPUNCTURE/ACUPRESSURE

Acupuncture is a practice that originated in China in which tiny needles are inserted at specific points on the body to relieve pain and cure disease. In acupressure, the practitioner applies pressure to the specific sites instead of inserting needles into the skin. When performed by a qualified practitioner, both of these methods can produce positive results. Many people report a reduction in pain and symptoms—and sometimes, complete relief.

ALLERGY ELIMINATION DIET

In an allergy elimination diet, you remove all suspect foods from your diet for two weeks. Suspect foods may include dairy, wheat, shellfish, and gluten. If no improvement is seen, you may still be eating foods that you are allergic to. Try to eliminate as many more foods as possible. When you are no longer experiencing any symptoms, add one eliminated food back to your diet. (Of course, if you know for sure that you are allergic to it, do not add it back.) If there is no reaction after two to three hours, that particular food should be safe to eat. Then, each week, add one more food back to your diet. This way, you should be able to determine which foods are causing the problem. Once you know which they are, be sure not to eat them at all or symptoms may return.

AROMATHERAPY

Aromatherapy is the practice of using essential oils—the distilled essences of plants, fruits, and flowers—to promote and enhance physical and emotional well-being. Essential oils can be inhaled from the bottle, applied to the skin in carrier oils, added to bathwater, used in therapeutic steam inhalations, and dispersed in the air with a diffuser. It's important to purchase essential oils from a reputable manufacturer to make sure that the products you buy are pure. Also, when purchasing aromatherapy products, such as candles, be sure that they actually contain essential oils and no synthetic fragrances.

BIOFEEDBACK

Biofeedback is a treatment technique in which a person receives immediate feedback on unconscious or involuntary body processes to eventually gain control over them. Clinical biofeedback is often used successfully for pain management, muscle movement and control, and circulatory dysfunction. If you think biofeedback might help your condition, seek out a trained biofeedback therapist in your area. Depending on your needs, the therapist may recommend a course of several sessions in addition to at-home practice.

DOUCHING

A douche is a preparation of water usually mixed with a healing substance that is jetted into the vagina using a special device. Commonly used to simply cleanse the vagina, douches can also be used for healing purposes. Store-bought douches often contain harsh chemicals and should be avoided. You can purchase a device specifically for douching at your pharmacy and can prepare a natural solution at home, using vinegar and water, unprocessed plain yogurt with live cultures, boric acid and water, or a few drops of tea tree oil and water. Douche only occasionally, as frequent douching can upset the balance of healthy bacteria normally present in the vagina.

EXERCISE

Exercise is important for a healthy body, but many people do not get enough regular exercise. A strong, toned body is less susceptible to infections and recovers quicker. Exercise also relieves stress, which strengthens the immune system. When regular exercise is recommended, it doesn't necessarily mean that you should run laps or lift heavy weights. Exercise can simply be taking a long walk, climbing stairs, participating in a sport, or any number of other physical daily activities. If you haven't exercised for a long time, start slowly and increase your activity when you feel you can handle it. Before starting any type of exercise program, check with your doctor.

Fresh Fruit Diet

Fresh Fruit Diet

If you are suffering from a weakened immune system, a temporary diet consisting of fresh fruit can help to strengthen it. While on this diet, you eat only fresh fruit for two to three days. You can also juice the fruit occasionally, but the fiber that you get from the whole fruit is important. Dark-colored fruits are best, and although they are not fruits, dark green leafy vegetables are also good to eat. While you are on this diet, you can continue taking your regular supplements. Be sure to drink six to ten glasses of water daily while on this diet to prevent changes in your bowel movements. When you go off this diet, you should add other foods back in slowly.

Homeopathy

Homeopathy

Homeopathy is a time-tested practice of treating a disorder by administering small doses of a remedy that would produce the symptoms of that disorder in a healthy person. Homeopathy has become a well-respected alternative to conventional medicine. Homeopathic remedies for virtually everything from acne to warts can be found on the shelves of nutrition centers and health food stores. Moreover, homeopathic practitioners who tailor remedies to your specific needs are becoming increasingly more common.

MASSAGE

Body massage can be described as the manipulation of soft tissue for therapeutic purposes. Massages can successfully treat illnesses brought about by stress, such as tension, aches and pains, insomnia, and headaches, all of which are accumulated in the course of daily life. The pain-relieving effects associated with skin stimulation and increased temperature that result from a massage help induce relaxation, both mentally and physically. It is very popular today to regularly attend a spa, where any number of different massages from shiatsu to Swedish are available. However, trading massages with a partner or friend is less costly.

MEDITATION

Meditation is the practice of sitting calmly and emptying one's mind of day-to-day concerns and concentrating on one specific thought or *mantra,* a word or phrase that embodies an ideal or guiding principle. When practiced regularly—for anywhere from five minutes to a half-hour each day—meditation can help induce relaxation and promote clearer thinking. Meditation centers are becoming more common, but you can meditate anywhere—even on a long line at the bank. Also, guided meditation audio tapes are widely available.

SAUNAS

A sauna is a steam bath in which water is poured on hot coals to produce steam. Many gyms, health spas, and resorts have a room specifically for this purpose. Some people even have them installed in their homes—usually at a great expense. The temperature in these rooms can be quite high, so anyone who is ill should avoid them or discuss their use with a doctor. In relatively healthy people, saunas promote relaxation and help cleanse the body of toxins because the humidity and high temperatures promote sweating. The time spent in the sauna should be limited to about ten to twenty minutes, and should be followed by a shower.

TAI CHI

Developed in ancient China, tai chi is a type of meditative exercise. In this system, a series of preset movements are performed slowly and fluidly. While practitioners may make it look easy, it does require quite a bit of effort. The benefit is that it has an overall relaxing effect on the body and mind. Centers that have tai chi classes are becoming more common. Some martial arts studios and health clubs may also offer tai chi classes. While it's a good idea to learn the techniques from an instructor, tai chi videotapes are available so that you can practice in your own home.

YOGA

Yoga is a system of poses that developed in ancient India. It induces relaxation and improves the flexibility of your muscles. Presently, there are many different styles of yoga. If you are interested in this system, it's a good idea to research what types of yoga are available in your area and determine which is right for you. While certain philosophies are often attached to this practice, it can be performed without this connection. Many health clubs and centers offer daily yoga classes. Once you learn the poses, you can easily practice at home.

About the Author

Earl Mindell, R.Ph., Ph.D., is an internationally recognized expert on nutrition, drugs, vitamins, and herbal remedies. He is the author of more than fifty books, including the *New Vitamin Bible, Prescription Alternatives, Soy Miracle, New Herb Bible, Anti-Aging Bible, Peak Performance Bible,* and *The Diet Bible.* He is a registered pharmacist, master herbalist, and a professor of nutrition at Pacific Western University in Los Angeles. He conducts nutritional seminars around the world and lives in Beverly Hills, California.